AH, FOOD, WHY DO YOU TROUBLE ME SO MUCH?

Tuvevun Publishing
Tuvevun@gmail.com

ISBN: 978-1-7343734-0-0 (print)
ISBN: 978-1-7343734-1-7 (ebook)

Ordering Information:

Special discounts are available on quantity purchases by corporations, associations, and others. For details, contact Tuvevun@gmail.com

AH, FOOD, WHY DO YOU TROUBLE ME SO MUCH?

A simple and easy-to-use
meta-diet method for changing
your relationship to food

Or

14 mental and emotional steps you need
before you take one more bite

Todd Nyholm

CONTENTS

AUTHOR'S NOTE

For ease of use, this book is written in four sections:

Section 1 (Chapters 1-3) covers how the Nytality Method came about, the ideas basic to this work, and why you should use this method. You'll also find a short list explaining the principles.

Section 2 (Chapters 4-19) describes the principles in sequence. It also provides information to help you understand them and allow them to change the programming you have about yourself, food, and why you eat the way you do.

Section 3 (Chapters 20-21) includes a synopsis of each principle along with a little bit of explanation for those looking for a skeleton version to get started right now. You'll also find a plan to revisit more detailed explanations later. It concludes with a farewell to the reader to encourage you on your way and gives you a few things to think about on your path to changing your relationship to food.

Section 4 provides an addendum of information to help you if you are struggling to accomplish your goals with relation to food, diet, vitality, and health. It also includes a few concepts that encompass more than food. These concepts are still fundamental for getting the most out of the Nytality Method. They will become more important down the road, as more published works become available about the various elements of the system.

SECTION 1

CHAPTER 1

AH, FOOD, WHY DO YOU TROUBLE ME SO MUCH?

"All you have to do is live on broccoli and chicken breast and you will lose weight," says Super Fit Guy. I have heard this so many times. It has somehow become the golden rule of thoughtless diet advice. "It's so easy, just look at me! I was four pounds overweight and I'm down six, so just do what I did."

"Well, what do I do if the chicken breast and broccoli diet gives me unbearable heartburn, stomach cramps, and constipation?" I say to Super Fit Guy.

"No, no, no. That doesn't happen. You're just lying to me and yourself. You have no character."

"No, really, I've been in terrible pain."

"Yeah, okay, whatever, you're lazy and weak. I get it, just, you know, whatever, go see the doctor."

So I went to the doctor.

"Doctor, I'm having problems with diarrhea and constipation and sometimes heartburn," I say, with embarrassment.

"Ah, well, sadly you have bad genetics. Just live on Pepto, Imodium, and Pepcid for the rest of your life," says the well-meaning MD.

"Well, can we fix the problem?"

"Nope, you are just broken," replies the physician, sounding irritated.

"Will diet help?"

"Not really, no, just get some stock in Imodium," quips the doc as he leaves the room.

These might not have been the way the conversations ran verbatim, but they were pretty close. They left me feeling really bad about myself.

❦

"Don't worry, this diet works for everyone. Just eat only uncooked veggies and fruit, and then drink Diet Coke," says Diet Fad Gal.

"I've been doing that and I haven't gone to the bathroom in the last two months. What do I do now?"

"Well, do you get up at 5:00 a.m.?"

"No, I'm usually asleep then."

"Oh, I see. That's why this diet isn't working for you. You're just lazy and fat."

I've actually had this conversation too, even if I've plugged in a little exaggerated humor. They're difficult for me even to recount. What do you do when even the authority figures like doctors don't have an answer for you and instead attack your character and personality?

We need an approach to diet that isn't one size fits all and perhaps one in which the main principle of the diet isn't just that you're lazy, fat, and have no character or willpower. How do you build incredible willpower when every diet you've tried has failed? Maybe you've even gotten bigger and you have no vitality left after eating foods that don't give you the nutrition you need. Or what about when you are emotionally depleted from having to defend yourself and use the energy from food as an emotional buffer to stop personal attacks?

How do we begin to dig ourselves out of this trap? How do we start to change the discussion on this very important aspect of our lives for ourselves? How do we discover our motivations, habits, and emotional and mental downfalls with regard to food?

How do we do it in such a way that doesn't make life lose all meaning and interest?

Ultimately, this is not a book about diets. This is a book about discovering and working with your relationship with food in real time. It's written in a way that allows you to bounce around and take what you need from each chapter while beginning to build synergies with the rest of the principles. You don't need to read them in order or apply them all at once. Take whatever works and use that, and then add a new principle and use that until it works. Do this until you have a workable program that fits you and your life.

I kept the book short so you can use it as a manual for action, personal reflection, and accomplishment. I hope you use it to make some real, sustainable changes in your relationship to food and your daily life.

Emotional wounds

It's important to begin by pulling back the layers on why we do what we do when it comes to food and drink and in terms of "feeding" our lives. We are so full of habits and motivations from all the way back to when we were kids. The thing is, we were often learning by very poor example. We've been taught to eat in excess. We've been taught to eat nonnutritious food. We've been taught to console and reward ourselves with the same sugar-laden treats. We pay no attention to ourselves or our food when we eat, and then we wonder why it's so difficult to make the changes that we need.

For many of us, the subject of food and eating has left knots of emotional wounds. Worse, we don't examine these wounds with empathy, sustained attention, and due diligence. Our cultural narrative tells us that people struggling with their weight are morally, emotionally, and personally bankrupt. This is a much bigger story than we think, than we have been told, than we have been sold. We need to look under the hood to investigate the motivations and unconscious habits that we have used to get through our lives with our relationship to food.

This book is meant to be your first step in that direction. It's meant to be used as you eat, to help you understand what you are doing and why, and help you make changes in your personal relationship to food and diet. It's written for all types of people: Whether you are an intellectual, emotional, or physical person, there's material for each viewpoint. Please look at this as a journey, and don't torture yourself because you didn't accomplish your goals by last Tuesday at noon.

I recommend you keep this work quiet. Make the changes you need to make and show the world rather than talking about it and getting massive resistance to what you are trying to achieve. Much of the time this resistance is meant to somehow help you, but in reality it makes things much more difficult.

Maybe you've heard you're just "thick-boned," or that "our family is just really big." It may seem true but how often is your bad health simply a result of the bad habits and negative culture you unconsciously learned from your family, not your actual genetics? There is such a strong series of cultural viewpoints on this subject that it can be easy to get confused and to feel attacked when you are trying to make a positive change in this area of your life.

Instead of a diet, what I want to share with you here is a method for changing the concepts of food and eating that you now hold in your internal world. I want to make how you eat, why you eat, when you eat, and what you think of food and your body conscious acts and therefore malleable to conscious change. For most people, their behavior with food is almost entirely unconscious. They don't know that they eat to celebrate because their parents taught them to do so; they don't know that they reach for the proverbial "heartbreak ice cream" because they saw it displayed and rewarded in their favorite sitcoms again and again.

Why diets fail

Diets fail because people have not changed the underlying mental, emotional, and physical programing that drives their behavior.

There are plenty of good diets out there, but they will be sabotaged if you don't consciously address the underlying coding of how you think, feel, and sense food and eating as a concept. Trying to change an internal problem with external force isn't the most effective way to create change, and sometimes you think you are getting something done when you aren't working in the right place to make an effective change.

A wonderful place to start is simply to ask yourself, "Why do I eat?"

What does that question bring to mind? Don't worry too much about the answer at first. Just asking the question will begin the process. We want to begin to gently overhaul your concept of food. We also want to question how we feel about food.

Don't dwell too much on the why for now; just getting into the questions will begin to change your inner world if you do it diligently and with sincerity. Shine some light on the feelings you have about food. Ask yourself this now and write down the answer: **How do I feel about food and diet?** Take your time with this question, and when you've written your response, consider these questions:

- Is your answer generally positive or negative?

- Does your answer make you want to run and hide or give you feelings of anger?

- Does it make you feel strong and powerful or weak and broken? Something else?

Any answer is fine for now. Just see what comes up and make some notes about it.

Finally, we will think about how sensations of food drive our behavior. We will look under the hood of how your body works with food. For now, think about these questions:

- Do you ever eat to actively change the chemistry of your body? For example, do you chug down five Red Bulls to stay awake for class?

- Do you crave salt in the afternoon?

Consider all the sensations that lead you eat. For example, you might eat a whole bag of pistachios because you like how it feels to shell the nuts and chew as you watch *Keeping Up with the Kardashians* or the newest episode of *The Walking Dead*.

This chapter gave you some idea of where we are headed. I hope you will begin to look at this as a journey, a ride into new territory that can help you in your relationship with food. Again, there are many good diets out there, but maybe it's time we took back our power over how we eat and work with food.

A diet can't make us feel the love we didn't get as children. It might not fix a chemical imbalance caused by a damaged microbiome and long-standing health problems. But changing our relationship with food can change how well we live and feel each day. So buckle up and get excited as we begin our journey to discovering your own reasons for eating or not eating and giving you some tools to regain the vitality, body, health, and life of your dreams.

CHAPTER 2

WHERE AND WHY?

To begin, I want to tell you some of my story and how it led to the Nytality Method. I'll do this even though I am fairly anxious about the reaction I will get because it's important for you to know.

When I was quite young, I did exercises and meditations that made the world and myself feel a little different and more importantly, gave me some conscious control over my inner life. As I grew older and the enforced socialization of school began, I was forced to the "realization" that I was not supposed to be able to control my mind, emotions, and energies that way. So I walled that part of myself off to make sure I could fit in and be a "good boy." Those early ways of doing things are the origins of the Nytality Life Method.

I've had health problems for as long as I can remember. Even at two or three years old, I experienced stomach cramping, reflux, intestinal cramping, diarrhea, and constipation.

Other kids mocked me. And my teachers didn't believe in my symptoms. When that happens, you naturally learn to shut up and take it.

I struggled with tissue pain, joint pain, never-ending extreme exhaustion, blocks in my ability to think clearly, and the somewhat natural depression and anxiety that follows all of that. Family doctors and nurses diagnosed me with IBS and said the other symptoms were in my head. They said I was just lazy and wanted attention.

So even though I was in constant pain and discomfort, I started to search everywhere for an end to the suffering I felt. That really stoked my natural interest in philosophy and useful ways of living. I remember spending hours in the library when I was 10 years old searching for ancient information on health, spirituality, martial arts, philosophy, yoga, ways of working with the mind, ways of working with the emotions, diet, massage, reflexology, acupressure, and so on. I stayed up all night trying to find answers, and to this day I still do. I felt pain on every level of my existence, and I was quite unwilling to just accept that fate.

Birth of the method

All of this is the genesis of the approach I eventually called the Nytality Life Method—many of the methods I had within me and even practiced as a child. Looking back, I know I was waiting for someone to teach them to me.

As I grew older, I got involved in martial arts. I went from school to school looking for someone who could do what was suggested in books about Asian martial arts. When I was 18, I found a teacher who could do those things and teach them. As fortune would have it, he was also an acupuncturist, a naturopath, and a homeopath. This was the first help I received that actually made a difference for me, even in the midst of some by-then rather intense cynicism and doubt. He helped me get through many problems and taught me things that have literally saved my life. There is no way to adequately thank someone who has had that kind of effect on your life, but let me say it here: I can't thank you enough, Doc. You have my utmost gratitude. You helped me keep going when there were times I didn't know how to keep going.

Even with the doc's help, I was still in pain, and I still hadn't found all of what my heart was desperately trying to find. It took me a lot more pain to realize I was looking in the wrong place. I had found the best of what I could find outside of me. The answer I desperately needed was inside me. It had been there since I was a child.

So I naturally started gravitating towards working in health-care. I learned massage, reflexology, Structural Integration of The Rolf Method, visceral manipulation, acupressure, and a few more physical types of therapies. I was trying to solve my own pain and give myself resources, but I was also pushed because I love helping people. I found many answers that have helped me along the way. Looking back now, the step-by-step methods were first formulated as a physical manipulation therapy and grew from that beyond my wildest imagination. Every day, I use the physical methods I put together with the ones I learned at the clinic.

My healing

As I got older, my health continued to decline. That led me to more doctors until I went to see a functional medicine doctor. He spent more than an hour with me after we had run some tests and said, "I think I know what has been ailing you all of these years." I had been bitten by a tick or some vector that had given me some nasty infections, probably, we estimated around the time I was five. That weakened my immune system and left me an easy target for some other interesting problems with parasites, fungi, and viruses. So we began to treat them. The fights with the infections have been extremely difficult, but over a couple years it began to make a difference.

For years, I struggled with my memory. But thanks to the treatment, I started to get memories back. I began to understand a great many things. I had experienced a couple of years of truly terrible sexual abuse and sadistic emotional manipulation by a neighbor when I was quite young, and as I went through the healing of the infections, I gained access to those memories. That helped me understand some odd snippets of memories I had and my reluctance to pull at the threads of those memories. In my efforts to heal myself, and through the development of my methods, I made myself strong enough to look at what happened. I got help from a wonderful counselor, and she and I diligently worked through it.

All of this healing, working through things, and being able to remember drew me to what I had somehow always known I needed to do in my time here, which was to finish developing these methods that were pouring out of me. My approach includes an abundance of methods based on a few dozen core principles which are meant to help you become aware of and work with various parts of you. There are physical, mental, and emotional methods, self-care methods, approaches to working with trauma, vitalizing methods, and more.

I have been relentlessly working on ways to help myself, and to help others work on themselves, so that we can change our inner worlds specifically. But these methods can also make our outer worlds more into what we want.

These methods have often shown up fully formed in my mind, like an itch. I can feel something in the back of my mind. And when I sit to look at them, they start to almost automatically download onto the page.

Simple but powerful

None of this is radical or horribly difficult to do. Most of it is similar to other methods out there, but it is interlaced with itself in a way that I think can help you on a few different levels at once. That interlacing and stacking effect has a profound effect on the usefulness of the methods, as well as helping them become more permanent in your experience.

I wrote this book for myself. I needed these principles, methods, examples, and lifestyle help as much as (or more than) anyone else. Life is short. I spent two years wondering every day if I was going to survive the health problems I had. Being ground down like that very much changed what I thought I was capable of: I have become much more comfortable with the idea of upsetting people and downright pissing a few people off. The visceral knowledge that I am going to die, and that I might die quite painfully, makes the idea of not doing what is most important to me in this life unbearable and unacceptable. In many ways, it's a bloody miracle I am here at all. I don't take that lightly. I want to make a few waves.

The NLM is legitimately the coolest thing I can possibly imagine. It is my great hope that it will touch you and your life in a similar way it has for me.

I chose to start with this specific book on food because day after day in my practice, I hear people talk about the difficulties they have with their health, their weight, their view of themselves, and their energy. And day after day I've heard myself say those same things.

I tried everything and wasn't able to find the answers I was looking for. In fact, a lot of what I found was mental and emotional attacks on the situation or the people struggling to find the answers that they needed. Everyone knows someone who eats total garbage in large quantities and doesn't exercise. How do they stay thin and somehow reasonably energetic? And my guess is, you also know a person or two who works hard on their diet and is trying to live on their treadmill but is still overweight and exhausted.

Clearly, people need to eat well and exercise appropriately to be healthy, vital, emotionally put together, and mentally sharp. But the results can be difficult to see if you don't give it enough time. Some people can go decades eating terribly, neglecting proper exercise, and living in anger. These people ignore any interest in or diligent activity towards building health or vitality and still "appear" to be the paragon of health. But with a long enough timeline, you will see them crash. Other people, from day one, struggle with exhaustion, weight problems, cravings, and depression. It's a massive disservice to write anyone off as just lazy. Naturally, however, if you aren't working to remedy that situation you are doing yourself a large disservice.

But that brings up a second problem: What if you are working on it but can't seem to get the results you want? One of the things I have found most distressing is how so many people who have hit the genetic lottery go into the health and fitness sector. They got there because it was the path of least resistance. They were always in the upper 10 percent of fitness, physical function, and energy and so they naturally gravitated towards that industry. That is wonderful if you want to see the top end of what a human can do in regard to their fitness, strength, endurance, physical beauty, and ability to stretch the limit of what a human is capable. But—and this is important to see—it is of no help in understanding the struggles of the bottom 10 percent.

This is not an attack on the people for whom health and fitness come rather naturally. On some level, it is like a talented musician trying to understand someone who is a bit tone deaf or a genius trying to understand someone who may be developmentally challenged. It is difficult to see clearly what isn't in your wheelhouse to begin with. That doesn't mean that it is impossible for these people to understand people who struggle. There are many who do a good job at closing that gap, but we need to acknowledge that it exists.

Some reasons why

Hormones, early childhood experiences, sexual or emotional abuse, infections, intestinal problems, emotional stability difficulties, diabetes, fibromyalgia, chronic fatigue, self-esteem issues, and a hundred other things play into how we understand food and fitness. To shrug people off as being just lazy is appalling. People are far more powerful than we think. We don't say this enough to each other: You are capable of great things. Don't stop moving forward; don't ever stop trying to find the way to the answers that you need. If there is one message I want to share at the beginning of this journey, it would be to decide now that you won't stop until you reach the answers you seek. Be quietly unstoppable. If you need at least one person to say it to you, here you go: You can do this. You have what it takes. The things you are capable of would absolutely blow your mind. Work in that direction, diligently over time, positively in your emotions, and seek solutions with an open mind.

This book is the first in a series that can help you improve in almost every area of your life. It will also generally help to answer a question that has been burning in my heart as long as I can remember: How do we live a life that is fulfilled so at the end of our lives we can say to ourselves—*that was exactly what I was looking for?*

Food is a wonderful place to start making a change in your life. "Food" is feeding every aspect of you and your life. There are many types of "food." In this book we will be looking more directly at the physical food we take into our bodies but you can apply the word "food" to many elements of your life. One of my teachers taught me years ago that food encompasses everything that you consume, including TV, movies, books, music, and even social interaction. This is a wonderfully useful principle.

Is what you are taking in nourishing you?

Use this right now with whatever you can get to work

This book is written to be used and to be used right now. This is meant to impact what you are doing right now and not simply to give you another thing to read and think about without creating action and some sort of change in your daily life. You could take any principle in the book and start with it. You should be able to open any page and find something you can work with, right now as you are. That being said, this method uses a ladder approach that brings the most out of the principles and later will be tied to many other NLM practices. The system ties the various parts of you together concurrently, so each method builds exponentially off the others. Each element is a stepping stone to improve yourself and your quality of life.

The next chapter puts your feet on the ground floor from which you will start the NLM. It is fundamental to everything else. Underlying these principles is the idea that you matter and that you want to treat yourself accordingly, consciously. And so off we go on this journey!

CHAPTER 3

LET'S THINK ABOUT WHY WE EAT

Sometimes, you need to address other problems first

If you use food to make life more bearable because you are in pain and suffering, then "dieting" can crush the pain-bearing effect the food has for you. Any of you who suffer, or have suffered, from chronic illness might know what I mean. Sometimes that latte is the only thing that dulls the pain.

That's a bit of an extreme example, but hopefully you can catch the meaning from the extremity of it. You need to replace "food as your only pleasure" with something else. If you really are only holding on to life right now because food feels good, don't stop that yet. Find something else to hold on to before you stop using food. Please get some help if you are in that place. There are many wonderful doctors and therapists who can help you. Remember, it is okay to switch medical professionals until you find someone who can genuinely help you. Do what it takes to hold on.

This is another reason to become conscious of our food motivations: We might answer the wrong question about why we eat the way we do if we're not fully aware. Giving chronic pain sufferers a diet of cucumbers and chicken to help them stop eating brownies is the wrong answer and it won't work. Their pain needs to be addressed so that the diet can go back to being about food and nutrition rather than about pain relief and lifting moods. Perhaps, this sounds obvious, but it is vitally important to consider the impact of pain on our behavior with food.

This work goes well beyond understanding your diet and body woes. It can yield great insight into your health and vitality in general. It can become a project of massive discovery. It can literally become a means of changing your life and direction. Food takes up a large amount of time, money, and effort. Despite all that, it rarely occupies the amount of attention it deserves.

Take some time now to make a list of the reasons you eat. Add to it over the next few weeks and months. Make your motivations clear to you.

How is your relationship with food working for you right now?

Most of this book is designed to lead you to ways to coax changes into your life. It's meant to plant seeds and have them grow for your use through repetition and application over time. This particular section, however, is meant to help you call yourself out. Naturally, for this to work you will need to be honest with yourself—but that can begin to set you free—free from all the garbage we tell ourselves in order to justify our behaviors, thoughts, and emotions. Remember, this is just you with you! There's no reason to be embarrassed or ashamed. Those emotions might seem useful, but they're actually helping you stay stuck in the past and keeping you locked in a deception about yourself: it's the lie that you will always be who you were or who you are right now.

Come at it from a beginner's mind and start with a fresh slate. You can always pick up that old stuff later, if you like. You are a human being with almost unlimited potential. Now is the time to make a change! Put aside the blame, shame, frustration, and anger.

From this fresh slate and new viewpoint, ask yourself these questions. You don't have to come up with long answers; the questions are just meant to clarify for yourself what your relationship with food is right now, as you get started. Some of these questions (and their answers) might be a little painful, but that's okay. They were for me too.

- In the broadest sense, how well is your relationship with food working for you? Answer however it makes sense for you—a scale from 1 to 10 or in a few words. A more complex answer is fine too.

- How often do you feel good, vital, healthy, and strong? Most of the time? Once a week? Only now and then? Almost never?
  o Have you ever felt vital, good, and healthy? How long has it been since you felt that way?

- To what degree is your current relationship with food moving you closer to feeling good, vital, healthy, and strong? Are you there? Nearly there? Confused? Very far away?

- Do you feel vital, good, healthy, and strong enough to make necessary changes in your life?

- What do you understand right now about the way food influences how you feel and think? Be specific! Don't just wave your hand and nod—what do you actually understand right now?

- And now, the biggest question: What kind of life do you want? What five words would you use to describe the life you really want to be living?
  - Is your relationship with food helping or hurting you as you pursue that life?

Earlier I said we want to coax these changes into our lives. We want to make changes that are sustainable and do it in ways that are enjoyable. Still, a good shock can help you change direction. Be brutally honest with yourself here. Get away from your pride and ego. Be brave. Address your true attitudes and beliefs. It's only from where you actually are that you can make a change. There is no shame or embarrassment in seeing where you are; in fact, it takes courage to really see yourself. This is just for you, privately; don't concern yourself with what others think. Don't let anything or anyone block your progress.

Now let's get a little more specific. Have you noticed that when you eat a big, greasy meal you feel lethargic, emotionally low, maybe even a bit depressed and mentally sluggish? Maybe you can remember a Thanksgiving dinner where after the celebration you could barely stand up? Of course, there are times you should celebrate and eat to your heart's content, but is that how you want to feel from your diet? Remember, diet comes from the Greek for "a way of life." Do you want to feel that way every day? After every meal? Imagine: If a meal can make you feel down like that, then the right way of eating can do the opposite! What would it be like to eat in a way that makes you feel energized, enthusiastic, cheerful, and mentally sharp? Now, imagine how much your life could change if you lived this way for a year—or even a decade! What you eat, how you eat, and in what emotional state you eat has a huge impact on your life and specifically on how you feel.

We get lost in diets that keep us from getting what we want and leave us starving ourselves of some of the greatest experiences life has to offer. What is it worth to feel full of life? No matter where you go, there you are in this body. The old phrase still rings true when so much of your experience of life is set for you by the body you are in.

You'll need to take a look at the truth. This is a really big step. It takes courage and some real heroic fortitude. If you are overweight, just be okay with seeing that truth. If you eat because it is the only pleasure in your life, be willing to acknowledge that. If you starve yourself because you are trying to meet some beauty standard, observe that. Once you can see what the problem is, you can take steps to address it. If you need help to see this clearly, please get the help you need. By definition this effort is a strength, not a weakness; a strong person does what is necessary and a weak person hides from it.

I applaud you for seeing the problem and being willing to take the necessary steps to get what you need. It's a huge sign of being awesome. It makes you genuinely a badass. You certainly have my admiration.

Make health, vitality, the body you would like to develop, and the life you desire the concepts around which you build guideposts for your relationship with food. Consider briefly how much this attitude alone could change how you see and view what you bring into your body! There are many ways to reach your goals, and I'm not going to tell you to never eat the things you love. This isn't a diet book, remember?

Have you found yourself eating and really wishing you weren't?

So often we just consider this to be a lack of willpower. And of course on some level, it is. But maybe it'd be more useful to address the desire directly and not just resist it with willpower. Willpower eventually runs out and then you're bound for a crash. If you haven't changed the internal drive for the food or behavior, it will come out when you are exhausted, emotional, or even just bored.

Now let's move beyond the question of what to eat and think about the specific scenario in which you're eating, even as you're wishing you weren't. Ask yourself these questions each time you find yourself in this situation:

- When this happens, why are you eating? When do you eat most frequently like this?

- What are you getting out of the food and the meal?

- How are you eating? Be specific! Are you usually on the couch? Standing in the kitchen? Driving? Mindlessly putting food in your mouth in front of the computer? Standing in front of the open refrigerator in the middle of the night?

- When you're eating like this, with whom are you most often eating? (Maybe you're usually alone when you eat like this. That's okay. Note that down too.)

If you really want to gain better control of your relationship to food, it's essential to dig deep and examine all the reasons, motivations, and how-tos of what you're doing, and that includes what's happening when we choose to eat. We don't consciously see that food is building our lives, supporting it, interacting with it, changing our emotions, thoughts, relationships, self-esteem. It can create illnesses, poverty, our wealth, our drives, and everything else that affects our experience of life.

What do you know about how and why and when you eat?

This next set of questions can help you to get a picture of how food is affecting your daily life and your experience of it. Take the time to work through these questions on paper to help clarify for yourself this area of life, which can be so routine it doesn't get any conscious attention. Take yourself seriously, here; this project is yours and the time you spend now will pay off.

- Does what you eat affect your experience of the day? Think through your days or the rhythm of your weeks. Maybe the coffee and donuts at the Monday morning staff meeting make you crash midmorning. Maybe Mondays are already tough because you let yourself be out of control over the weekend. Do you skip breakfast? Snack all afternoon? Pull out all the stops because "it's the weekend?"

- Do you live on caffeine? Why?

- Does food kind of control you? This is probably true for a great many people. What does this mean for you?

- Do you eat food out of the compulsion for that specific food rather than for the vitality and enjoyment food gives you in terms of your life? Sweets and salty foods are common examples, but some people are drawn toward the foods of their childhood. For you, which foods have the most powerful effect in this way?

- If you had to describe your current relationship to food in five words, what would you use? What words would you rather use?

- Pause for a moment and think about the life of your dreams. Really bring it to life in your mind. Make it real and vivid.

- What foods do you eat now that are damaging your ability to reach the life of your dreams?

- What food, drink, and habits with food would help you accomplish the life of your dreams? Why?

These questions may seem simple, but they are designed to help make things you probably already feel or know more conscious so you can work on this part of your life directly.

This is why I encourage you to take the time to reflect on these questions and write down your answers. You can "know" something without thinking much about it, but when you have to actually put it into words, you can learn important things that will help you. Often, we can miss things that need diligent attention because we think we already have it down. As you work through this book, if you find yourself stuck or not getting the results you want, come back here and explore the questions in greater depth.

How do we begin to change our relationship with food?

There are three steps to changing the way you relate to food:

1. The first step is to make as much of what you are doing, thinking, feeling, and sensing conscious to yourself. So much of what we do becomes habitual, and you need to be able to see those senses, actions, and thoughts clearly. We want to understand our motivations and habits, so step one is to begin to be present while you eat. Start by eliminating distractions while you eat. Turn off the TV, put away your phone, try not to have deep philosophical conversations. Focus on the food in front of you. How does it smell? How does it taste? How does it feel in your mouth? How long did it take to make?

   This might suck at first. It's a surprisingly big change to not eat while watching football, discussing the events in Washington, or reading a good book. Start slowly and work towards being present, being in your body, and being engaged with yourself more and more over days, weeks, and years. The idea is to become conscious of what you think, feel, and sense while you eat, not to become a hermit. Start patiently and work to maintain and build a little personal practice over time. You don't need to be alone, you just need to be present and paying attention. This will get easier over time.

   Maybe start with eating a cookie by yourself. Eat the cookie and see what you experience. Be curious. Notice what you are thinking and feeling, and what your body is sensing.

For now, don't make any judgments about these sensations. Judgments will only knock you out of the moment. The whole point is to be present and not run from it. Take the time and attention to build this new skill. It is worth way more than I can get across right now. You've got this. Go do that right now.

2. The second step is to begin to articulate for yourself what your goals are. What goals do you want your relationship with food to lead you towards? This needs to be personal. Don't list what you think you should do but instead what actually motivates you to make some changes. "Hot enough to attract any partner I want" might be more motivating to you right now than, "Because I guess I don't want a heart attack." Choose something that lights a fire. Script it to make you want to live more. How about something like, "I want my body to stop hurting," or "I would feel good about myself if I change this about myself." Ultimately, it needs to be about you and only you. What is your reason? What makes you feel more vital and alive?

3. Once you know what your goals are, visualize them for yourself. See them as real and vivid. Feel them all the way down to your bones. Then you can bring them up at will and—here's the important part—you can bring them up right before you eat. Wouldn't you want to see where you are heading? Seeing something you want and moving yourself towards it can bring passion to your life. Don't neglect this.

Naturally, these goals can simply be inspiring body goals. You can work and dream to transform your body in the way you wish. They can be other kinds of goals too: Promotions at work, vacations, education, inspiring your family, feeling vital, restoring your health, gaining muscle, sleeping better, developing better emotional control, building developmental skills. The possibilities are almost endless. Make this work for you. It should stir your soul. It should make your nerve endings quiver. It might take a while to get to that level, so just start with what works for you here and now and as you are. Know that you can change course successfully when you need to.

This is a much, much bigger start than you think. Take your time and enjoy this part of the process so it can be sustainable. If you enjoy it, you are much more likely to continue.

In a very real sense we are trying to set ourselves free: Free from compulsive eating, habitual emotions, and thoughts, and free from the chaos in our lives. In many ways we've become enslaved by our habits and ways of living that don't meet our best interests and desires. Set yourself free! Take control of your life. Learn to feed yourself and your life consciously with food.

Why so many questions?

You'll notice as you read this book—and almost everything I write—that I ask you questions without overtly telling you what to think. There are lots of questions in almost every chapter of this book. I want you to find some answers for yourself and to wake up to some new ways of doing things.

You may feel some distress as you're working through these questions. What you're feeling is normal as you discover new things about yourself. This pain of waking up has its usefulness to you, your life, and to helping you reach your dream life. There is no free lunch;

CHAPTER 4

WHY THIS METHOD?

This method gives you a system you can use right now to help you understand food as a principle and the ways in which food—and your relationship to it—dramatically affects your life. It will help you dig out for yourself how you got to this relationship and find a new way to live the life you dream about without being shackled to diets and chasing the food fads being sold to you.

Rather than relying upon massive willpower and resisting your inclinations and desires, this method will help you dig into your "food operating system," understand where you are coming from, and then give you a gentle but diligent means of rewriting that software—all while you eat.

This method works best when applied diligently, with your full attention brought to it regularly. This book is small enough that you can take it with you and use it whenever you might need it. It's meant to be an uplifting and motivating companion along the way rather than something to be read and left on the shelf. We can't always have a helpful friend to eat with, but this can be a little reminder along the way. Sometimes it's reassuring to know you aren't alone in the boat when the stormy seas feel like they are surrounding you.

This work builds on itself but each principle can be used on its own

The steps to the Nytality Method are quick to perform, relying much more on diligent application and repetition than on a forceful change in what you are "allowed" to eat. Think of it as a way to make sure that what you eat feeds all parts of you.

Each of the following chapters explains one of the basic principles. They will assist you in discovering why you eat, why you are eating right now, and how well your way of eating is working for you. Some of the steps will address how to understand food in a way that will nourish you. They will also help you see how food "feeds" your entire life. Embedded in some of the principles are ways to help you remember and apply what you already know about food and nutrition to what you are doing daily with your diet. We are all trying to get the most out of our time here and to feel the best we can while we are here. This method and the rest of the NLM are designed to help you do that.

Here are the 14 applied principles, and you'll see them reflected in the chapter titles to come:

- I eat to nourish myself and my life.

- Is there space needing to be filled?

- Stoke your metabolism.

- Have you considered what food brings you?

- Eat and drink foods that clean and cleanse you.

- Eat foods that aid digestion and movement.

- Eat a broad variety of nutrients, food groups, and colors within your veggies and fruit.

- Leave some space to digest your food and absorb what you drink.

- Pull vitality out of your food.

- What information are you taking in from your food and drink?

- What will you do with the energy (calories) from what you are eating?

- Eat foods that make you feel more emotionally in control and help you feel more like yourself.

- Consider how you would eat in order to think clearly, sharply, and concisely.

- Be grateful for the food you eat and that you have enough to sustain you.

Each of these steps stands for and is a means of reminding you of each principle and gives you a short phrase to remember during each meal. They distill the fundamental information presented in each chapter.

While the steps are organized with purpose, they can be used individually. Each is based on general principles systematically arranged within the whole system of the NLM.

Ultimately, they are a means of understanding different parts of you in relationship to each other. They have a compounding effect when applied in sequence. That being said, make them work in a way that fits into your life. This isn't a method carved in stone. It will work only when you bring it to life in your life.

This is for you

I want to say this again in order to help you apply this method successfully for you right now. At first, take anything from anywhere in this book, particularly if you like it or it catches your eye, and just make it work right here and now. Do it until it becomes familiar and almost does itself. You can stack the steps however you like, but fundamentally all of this rests on being able to take one thing and understand it, then apply it. Keep applying it without end. Add something, apply it without stopping. Do that over and over until you reach your desired goal. There is no special prize for trying to do it perfectly the first time, all at once. That's like trying to eat once and for all. Have fun with this. The only time you can change your life is right now, as you are and right where you are. You can do this, and this book will help! You don't have to work "hard" by making it difficult, but you do need to work diligently. Put your attention on it regularly and daily and you can't help but begin to make some changes. Start small, start often, and never ever stop. Take charge, without fanfare or gnashing of teeth, and do it right now. You are worth it.

CHAPTER 5

CHILDHOOD

This chapter is a little aside from the NLM process itself. In order to make the necessary changes, it's important to see that much of what you're doing in regard to food is not you, per se. You didn't decide it. You picked it up before you had the necessary faculties to decide its value or detriment to you and your health. This needs to be stated outright. Your feelings about food aren't you or yours and because of that you can change them. The power is in your hands, your heart, and your mind.

Where did your habits, thought processes, emotional habits, routines, and ideas come from regarding food, diet, health, body image, and vitality? A huge part came from your deeply impressionable years. At age three or four, you didn't have the tools you needed to question what your parents fed to you. It all went in unquestioned and unexamined.

Now is the time to examine it in a clear, concise, and purposeful way. Mentally pull it out, put it on the table, and look at it. Look at it in relation to what you need and want most in your life. Make it conscious to yourself so you can control the programming your mind is running.

As you do this, pay special attention to what you are feeling and what emotions are coming up. People like to think they are logical, methodical, and rational in their behavior and habits, but look more deeply and really feel what is going on within you. You are much more than your logical, rational mind. Do not throw out your logic; you need it to temper your emotions. But don't ignore your emotions either. Bring all of you to bear if you can and do it as consciously as you can.

Go back to your childhood mentally and feel

Now, think, feel, and sense what your childhood was like in general. Write stuff down so you can make it more real for yourself and come back to it later. If there is some crappy stuff back in your history and your story, try to work through it and sort out what happened in an intelligent, mindful way. Getting help from a therapist might be invaluable to you. Find what works for you. (Just like doctors, all therapists aren't the same.) If you're worried about the stigma of working with a therapist, don't let anyone know! In fact, this whole process might work better if you do it quietly, in the crucible of your own heart and the privacy of your own life. This is for *you*. This is *your* life, *your* body, *your* health, and *your* world.

I'm going to give you a long list of questions. They are simply meant to help you shed light on some long-standing habits, ideas, feelings, and thought processes that have been there so long it's hard to see when they started.

As you answer these questions, take time to remember what food was like for you as a kid. It is helpful to set aside some time to be alone and undisturbed so you can become almost meditative: For just a minute, stop and pay attention to your breathing. Get into your body, relax, and let your conscious mind settle down. Put your attention on your body and feel how everything feels *right here and now*. Our thinking tends to dominate our attention, but you can begin to break free of that domination by putting your attention consciously on your body. Use these questions as a springboard to explore your childhood exposure to food and eating.

What did you eat?

- What did you eat as a kid? What was a typical breakfast? Dinner?

- Was drinking alcohol modeled at every meal?

- Did your parents cook well?

- Did you eat a wide variety of foods?

- Was convenience food modeled at every meal?

How was food used?

- Did your parents console you with food? Reward you?

- Did your parents use food as a weapon?

- Was food made political?

- Was food used to manipulate or coerce you?

What were your dinners like?

- Did your family watch TV during dinner?

- Did your family fight at dinner?

- Was dinner time generally a nice time together or a stressful one?

- Did you dread this time or were you usually excited for dinner?

- Were you made to sit there for hours until you ate something inedible, poorly prepared, or something you just didn't like?

How did your parents describe your family's health history?

- How did your family describe their bodies? (Did your parents or family members describe your family as "big-boned" or as having lost the genetic lottery, for example?)

- Did your parents use weight to shame or guilt you?

- Does diabetes run in your family?

- Is there a history of alcoholism?

Meta-food problems derived from childhood

- Does answering these questions make you anxious and nervous?

- Does the entire subject of food, diets, and weight make you feel defeated because all the way back into childhood you have been struggling with it physically, socially, mentally, and/or emotionally?

- Can you still feel the sting of a family member, a trusted friend, or a medical professional's words about your character or worth as it relates to food and your body?

- On any level, do you feel like the size of your body determines your value as a person or your worth as a human being? What do you believe our culture says about how you look?

Remember, most people were doing the best they could, so just see clearly and decide what you would rather do than continue on with what was modeled for you. If things were done deliberately at your expense, then now is the time to look at it clearly, feel what you felt, and reframe the experience. Get help if needed; it's a sign of strength, not weakness. Someone strong does what is necessary to get the job done. You are in control now, you're not four anymore. Sometimes you have to tell yourself that. The past is done. The past is finished. Tell yourself it is done. This is more effective than you might think.

Work through this process at your own pace. Work with curiosity and act deliberately. Work until you can let go of the negativity that's holding you back now. Take the time you need, and take small steps that you know you can accomplish. Do it again and again until your goal is reached.

Again, and with the greatest compassion I can muster, if your past is too nasty to do it on your own, *get the help you need.* Then crush it! You are strong! You are capable. This is your life. This is your world. If you take conscious control of your inner world, then the world outside will follow. Look at it and make it conscious. Handle the emotions you feel, uncover the ideas that were modeled for you, and stay in your body to see how it reacts. See all of it dispassionately and pull it apart for yourself. Then choose new ideas, new emotions, and new physical actions and begin to consciously, deliberately, and playfully install those over time. You're just rewriting your own software. Make it an adventure! Make it a game, if you can. We all love games. Reward yourself as you make progress, even if that is just stepping aside and telling yourself, "I kind of kick ass. I did this, and it was difficult for me. Not everyone would do this. That speaks highly of me."

The material in this chapter may be a bit intense. If it seems particularly painful, there might be a lot of work to be done in this area. Do it with kindness and compassion for yourself. It can be easy to experience lots of negative self-talk when you do this kind of work and you may already be dealing with negative self-talk. It takes real courage to not beat yourself up but still get work done. With great respect I encourage you in this process—it takes real inner strength, and here you are, doing it!

CHAPTER 6

NOURISH MYSELF AND MY LIFE

Why do you eat?

Ask yourself this every time you eat. Ask yourself: Does this food nourish me and my life? Eat more of what does; eliminate more of what doesn't. If you do this small practice consciously and earnestly, allowing results to build on themselves, your relationship with food will change dramatically within a year. Your health and vitality will increase, not just because you believe it to be improving but because you changed your diet based on choosing food that gives you what you need. You can always do some research to see what foods are generally nutritious but check that against how you function with the food you eat.

First, develop a better understanding of why you eat. Food fuels your body, mind, and emotions. What you eat and drink fuels and influences every part of your experience of life. Consider how powerful that is! What you eat can also affect your sex life and your ability to enjoy it as you age. Your ability to enjoy life in almost every way is diminished by not taking care of your health and vitality!

Before you eat anything, say to yourself, "I eat to nourish myself and my life." When you say this before you eat, you are reprogramming your internal system. Refer back to the questions you answered in Chapter 3 any time you need to check in with yourself. Find what works for you here and now. What you learned from the answers to these questions can always be added to other diets and programs that fit with your new understanding of your needs.

At its essence and at its core, we take in food to nourish ourselves and our life. Of course, there are other reasons to eat, but check all of them against this one principle. This list of questions will help you apply the principle. Answer them honestly:

- Does this food nourish me and my life?

- Is this food adding to my health and vitality?

- Where is it taking away from these aspects of my life?

You don't need to be perfect; try to make it work for you most of the time. It's not about some painful regimen that makes life colorless and painful. You may find a strict approach useful as a resetting mechanism to change your tastes in food. And sticking to an intense, strict diet can give your taste buds and your body a useful rest.

This is so important as the base principle from which you'll work because it supports every other part of you and your life. If you can begin to live based on this principle, you can be reasonably assured that your life and relationship with food will be supportive of your mind, emotions, body, long-term success, long-term health, and any other short- or long-term goals you have. You may find this principle will spread into other areas of your life. What if you used the same principle in terms of how you think? (Is this thought nourishing me or my life, or is it destructive to me and my future?)

Add more of what nourishes, remove what doesn't. Be conscious and aware of what you are doing and why. Check your motivations and behavior about what you ultimately want, need, and desire. This is your life; start to act in accordance with that.

The applied principle for this step is to say to yourself, "I eat to nourish myself and my life."

CHAPTER 7

IS THERE SPACE?

How do you get back in touch with yourself about when to eat? Very often, people eat because it is lunchtime, because they are bored, because the game is on, because "everyone knows" you eat a big meal at six in the evening, because they had a killer commute, and lots of other reasons that actually have very little to do with food and its nutrition. It's helpful to have a conscious method to figure out why you are eating and whether this is a good time to eat for you and your bodily needs.

Before you eat, check in with yourself. Get into your body and feel what it is telling you. Then ask yourself these questions:

- Is there space that needs to be filled?

- Does it feel like my body needs or wants more food?

- Am I eating for another reason? Pause with this one and really check in with yourself.

I'm not saying to never eat for emotional or even mental reasons (for example, because I "know" everyone eats breakfast at 7:00 a.m.), but check in with your body first, every single time. You'll be surprised how much this simple practice can change your awareness of what your body needs. Asking this question recalibrates your attention.

What are you trying to fill or feed with what you are eating? Try to become aware of this as well. You may be trying to fill a hole in your heart rather than a hole in your nutrition. If you're eating to fill a hole in your heart, consider other ways, applied over time, to address that hole rather than using food to cover it. I'm not saying you need to abandon this coping mechanism completely—we all need ways of getting through difficult times—but finding a more direct way to heal that hole might do wonders for you and your life.

Remember, this whole method requires some profound inner strength to hear and see what is necessary. It takes courage to look where you don't want to look. What are you trying to fill, feel, or stop feeling by eating (or by not eating)? What might be a better long-term solution to accomplish that goal over time? (Again, getting some help might be useful for you. That's why counselors and therapists do what they do.)

As an example, when I was experiencing enormous pain every day as I was going through some of my treatments, I got in the habit of eating something sweet in the evening to give me something positive to look forward to. This was useful for a while but it made me feel more sick and tired.

So I began to work on some exercises and other aspects of the Nytality Method that made me feel more energetic. Those exercises began to feed me and helped me cope with the pain and deficit of proper neurochemistry. I look forward to teaching some of these aspects of the Nytality Method in future books. Ultimately, we want to begin to shift our perception of food and how it affects our bodies, making that the priority. If you haven't begun to consider the connection between your mind, emotions, and body, start now.

If you really want to help your mind and emotions work well, one of the best first steps is to address your body and nutrition adequately.

Learning to develop this skill with food and drink can have interesting ramifications for your entire life. Learn this aspect of discipline in a small, daily way and then you can extend it into the rest of your life, where you will need it in much bigger ways.

Filling yourself and your life only when there is space that needs to be filled is more important than you might think. We can be greedy for things we can't use, or that actively hurt us or get in the way of our most important goals, but we don't recognize it. Knowing when to stop is a skill you can develop. More is not always better, and sometimes more is so destructive it will completely destroy your life and your future or the lives of the people you care most about.

Let's be intentional with the word "discipline" since people misuse it as a substitute for punishment and enforced behavior modification. For the purposes of this book, I am using it only in the sense of how you *cut things* out that lead you away from what you are trying to create and for when you *add things* into your body, mind, emotions, schedule, and life in order to move closer to what you are trying to create.

Doing what you need to do—instilling discipline—isn't punishment, even if it hurts. It is the juice of champions, legends, and heroes. It is literally the stuff out of which a beautiful and powerful life is made. Be the hero.

The applied principle for this step is to ask yourself is their space open that I need to fill? Really feel your body. Take a breath. Then ask yourself is your body needing food right now?

CHAPTER 8

STOKE YOUR METABOLISM

B efore you eat, try to build the "burn." This concept became very important to me because I couldn't digest very well. Every phase of digestion was quite painful for me.

I struggled to break food down, pick up the nutrients, and eliminate the waste. I thought when everyone ate junk food they, like me, had intense cramping, diarrhea, and other such pains in the ass. Later, I learned I had a number of infections and problems that interfered with my ability to digest.

I've played with many ways to increase my digestion since I was a kid. One approach that will work well for everyone, but especially if you are working on rebuilding your health or when you are over-weight, is to do some isometric exercises right before you eat.

Isometrics are quite useful because you don't need to have any fitness level to begin with in order to get some benefit. Isometric exercises are things like wall push-ups, push-ups, squats, lunges, brisk walks, and stairs. They work to help stimulate your body. Do them just a little bit before you eat to prime the pump.

Put this into context for you and your life. Doing 100 push-ups before every meal might work for a few people but you might do much better if you just do a few isometrics in combination with a general weightlifting program. If you are starting from scratch, or fairly overweight, five wall push-ups per meal and five shallow lunges every single time you eat will help you begin to break inertia and create momentum. There is no telling how far that momentum can take you!

It also begins to change how you see yourself, and you may be surprised by the chain reaction that can set up in your inner life. Many people think they have to do some ego-aggrandizing number of exercises to make it feel "worth it" or "enough to make a difference," and since they can't do that, they do nothing at all. Things gets worse and worse, quickly. One repetition of any exercise daily over a year will break the slide into entropy, build a habit, start to build a little muscle, and set the stage for the next step, which will then help lead on to the next. Doing something every single day is of value in and of itself! You need to find a way to build yourself up or entropy; negative people and social media will break you down.

Because of the health problems I've had, I often could only do a few repetitions at a time, but I was always willing to do the few I could do. I kept silent about it to avoid ridicule and "tough love," but those few exercises allowed me to produce many things in my life no one else I know has done. Those few separated me from the pack in many ways. It's a different level of endurance and courage. Do not stop. Don't ever give up on yourself.

And as you break that inertia and social stigma, don't stop at one! Move on to two, do that until you are done. Then move on to four. If you do this for a few years, moving forward every day, soon you will be burying everyone who gave you a hard time. Do it as a lifestyle over decades and few people will keep up.

Use your experiences to grow

Some of you are furious, or angry. Perhaps, you've been belittled or mocked. If you want to shove it back in someone's face, do this quietly. Turn that anger into burning coals of motivation to set yourself free of whoever took shots at you, and you can get rid of whatever emotional button they pushed. You can take that anger and change it into a positive and motivating emotion. I recommend persistence and grit as motivating emotions and attitudes. Use that pain in your favor. In my estimation, I'm not sure there is much more that can make you a badass than starting from exactly where you are and kicking ass until you reach your goal. The further you have to go, the sweeter the accomplishment. Just start and don't stop. Don't ever, ever stop, even if you totally mess up one day. Just start again the next. That isn't a failure—that is the process. Without beating yourself up, just keep going, and going, and going.

Physical health is use it or lose it. It becomes more urgent the older you get. Walking is a great place to start, but ultimately you want to start taxing your musculature and putting weight-bearing pressure on your bones. If you are already in better shape, find your starting place, then push and test yourself. Grow by learning to push your boundaries. For Michael Jordan, five wall push-ups are not going to stoke his metabolism, but maybe 60 push-ups and 50 squats would do the job for him. Add this to whatever exercises you already do.

Please be careful to take care of your health. Ask your doctor about any exercise or exercise program you do.

Weight lifting and bodyweight exercises can be a valuable set of tools to speed up metabolism. You don't need to become Arnold Schwarzenegger, and you don't even have to worry about what you look like. The idea is to build your muscles creating a strong system that can help regulate your metabolism and hormones.

There are more ways than ever to approach this in your daily life: Gyms, workout groups, videos, Instagram, YouTube, websites, home weights, and books about weightlifting exercises are all available. Find what works well for you and run with it.

Remember, even one a day starts things moving and changing more than is easily perceptible. Then move to two after you break the inertia. Remember what you want to accomplish. See yourself there now, where you want to be. Have fun with it, don't make it life-or-death serious, and coax yourself forward. Take some pleasure in the work; if you enjoy some of it, you will be able to go further in the long run. This isn't about testing your willpower but about accomplishing something long term.

If you are already crushing it in weightlifting, high intensity interval training, or some other form of intense workout, you probably don't need this. Instead, you want to consider in the long run how you are burning calories and keeping your metabolism up through your general workout cycles. Timing your workouts to get the best result on your metabolic burn is key.

Turn up the heat. Use the necessary tools to stoke the fire in you.

The applied principle for this step is to use some activity in your life to build up your metabolism.

CHAPTER 9

GET THE MOST OUT OF YOUR FOOD: CHEW WELL

We eat depleted food while drinking sugar-loaded drinks, we eat in our cars, we eat while we are fighting with our spouse, and then we wonder why we feel exhausted, depressed, frustrated, sluggish, slow, and full of indigestion. We then curse our bodies for breaking down rather than appreciating the miracle work our bodies have done to keep us going for the last 50 years. Maybe now is the time to rethink and replace this approach. Your life is powered by your food. Your emotions and your ability to think clearly are influenced by your food, as well. Have some fun figuring how to build yourself up with the right foods.

We know about the nutrients we take from our food: Proteins, carbohydrates, fats, minerals, vitamins, and fiber are many of these substances. But can you see that you use food to power your life? Really consider this for a moment: Your life is powered by what you are eating and drinking and the oxygen from your breath. What kind of life do you want to have? A Twinkie-powered life (Twinkies aren't bad, they are just low-power food) or a life powered by food that is better able to power the life you want? Ask yourself: what foods would allow you to live the life you want?

Have you noticed some types of foods help you to think more clearly?

By contrast, some foods may muddy your thinking or gum up your physical works. This could be because foods stripped of their essential building blocks are high on refinement, farther from their source. And they are loaded with chemicals designed to make you want more, whether you want to eat or not. We all love our snacks, treats, conveniences, and sweets, but consider what would help you think clearly and sharply. What foods lead you to the life you want?

Snacks or treats aren't bad or evil, but using the intelligence within you, ask yourself what is leading you to more life. How often do you want to eat foods that lead you towards exhaustion, sluggish thinking, pain, and potentially disease?

Food doesn't just have a physical effect on us, of course. You may have noticed that some foods make you feel good emotionally and others drag you down lower and lower.

Some allow you more emotional control while others seem to take emotional control from you. Think of how you feel when you've had too much caffeine or too much sugar. Your decisions become rash. You may be quick to anger or have laughing fits.

Or put it this way: Imagine starting a fire in your fireplace using wood full of odd chemicals. Where would those chemicals end up? Maybe they are useful to start the fire quickly or maybe they even turn the fire into fun and unusual colors, but what happens to the fireplace over time? What is released into the air? What waste will we have to throw out later?

Remember, you are changing your relationship to food. The food you eat powers your life on a fundamental level. The quality of your life will, on some level, reflect the quality and quantity of the food you eat. Consider that your brain is also powered by the food you eat! When you eat, pause and consider that your life is built from what you are eating at that moment. Just keep this in mind for a minute or two and let it percolate. Given time, you might see that your appetites and your interests in food change.

Also, consider how you get what you need from food. Ultimately, it has to be broken down, assimilated, and excreted. Chewing enough can be essential for this process, especially if your digestion is compromised. Taking the time to chew properly will allow your body to pull out what is needed from the food. We also don't want to over-chew; we have stomach acid for a reason. Try to find the sweet spot for you by finding the right amount of food to take in and a pleasant amount of chewing. (Paying attention to this will also help you eat more mindfully!) This step is essential if your digestion is a bit poor, if you tend to gobble food with no regard to your ability to digest and process the food, or if you tend to eat in a hurry. Take time to eat. Your body needs certain conditions to function properly. Take the time to give it what it needs so your body can give you what you need.

Take a vitality inventory

Food is part of what creates the currency of life. For ease and for a simple term, I am calling that currency vitality. The way you eat will, in part, determine how much and what kind of currency you have to spend. Keep this in mind while you eat. How will this food affect how much currency I have to spend on my life?

Take stock of how much vitality or energy you have each day. This can be more useful than you might think! Many cultures have some kind of concept for "life energy." Think about the Chinese qi or France's élan vital.

If the concept of some kind of nebulous energy bothers you, then think of cellular energy derived from chemical reactions built from food, breathing, and hormones. While I think there is more to it than that, it is certainly true that those physiological, chemical reactions are happening and they provide you with a certain amount of resources with which to work.

Creating some kind of scale or metric for yourself can help you ascertain what gives you vitality. If you keep track, you can begin to see what helps you build vitality in your life and what drains it. Be careful of foods and drinks that seem to give you immediate energy.

The applied principle for this step is to chew well and thoroughly.

CHAPTER 10

CLEANSE AND CLEAN

Your system is intricately put together to accomplish many feats and withstand many hardships. Your body's ability to keep running and going even when you're eating garbage is incredible. Think about it: if you tried to run your car on the equivalent energy source of, say, three donuts, a Coke, and a three-day-old taco, it would sputter and die within a few days.

We want to take better care of our machinery so it works the way we want it to. Food and drinks that clean the system help to make that possible. As one of my teachers used to say, would you clean your Ferrari with Coke? Would you wash your clothing with coffee? Would you rather scrub them clean with a greasy piece of pizza or with a crunchy celery stick? I'm not saying never have pizza and Coke again, but we want to change your overarching thought processes and feelings about food. We want to start considering when and how to clean and cleanse our system with what we eat and drink. We want to start implementing habits that regularly include food that will have the effects we want and to avoid foods that take away from what we need and desire.

Have you noticed that when you eat a lot of junk food, slowly, almost imperceptibly, your thinking gets a bit off? How do you feel after you've had a three-day junk food bender? Or a real alcohol bender? Can you feel that clogging up of your system and your general functioning? It's like somehow your body is working so hard to deal with the processing of food that the resources you need to think well are missing.

Perhaps, you are young enough, or your digestion is almost perfect, and you don't notice this yet, but someday it will catch up with you. It eventually becomes important to realize how food affects you and your life. Your emotional state determines so much of your experience of life! It also determines a great deal of how much you will be able to accomplish.

You'd want to give yourself the right resources to have the life and body of your dreams. Food and drink (anything you have taken in, really) are your resources in real life. What can you build with what you take in? Or more specifically for this point, what effect is what you are taking in having on you, your emotions, your thinking processes, your vitality, and your overall life?

Here are some specific questions to ask yourself:

- How much clean, fresh water do you typically drink in a day?

- Do you eat an appropriate amount of veggies to help your system run clean? (How many servings did you eat yesterday?)

- Did you eat food with enough fiber to help keep moving things out?

If you've been living off of foods with lots of flavor enhancers, you're going to struggle to find foods without them tasty. You've been programmed to eat more junk food by manufacturers who artificially make food taste better. You might need time for your taste buds, body, emotions, and mind to adjust away from the chemicals used to add or boost flavor.

After you do, you might be surprised how sweet carrots are and—I can't believe I'm going to say this myself—how good broccoli can taste. When your taste buds have been blown out by super orange cheesy flavor enhancers, it's hard to get the flavor out of more subtle foods. Once you have everything back in perspective and in context, you can still splurge on your favorite snack foods but in a more intelligent and beneficial way. This is one reason eating foods that clean and cleanse you is so important. These foods will help clean these chemicals out and get you back to a more sensitive capacity to taste and to a more evenly functioning digestion.

It is common for authorities to give specific recommendations about the amount of vegetables, fruits, proteins like meat and fish, and grains one should eat during a given time. And in general, most people could use fewer grains, more vegetables, smaller meat proportions, and a general reduction in sugar consumption.

But the variety of diets that people can and do make work for their goals is much broader than would make specifics in this method useful. This method is designed, in part, to make how you feel a much bigger part of the picture than simple prescriptive guidelines might suggest.

So we go into how we feel directly and begin to work from there. This is a grand experiment in changing how you eat by observing how food makes you feel now and how eating that way makes you feel over time. You might be surprised how much information you can pick up by paying attention to this and how that can be a wonderful guide for building a diet that serves you and your needs.

Consider your diet as a whole: Do you have enough cleansing food and drinks to keep things working well? How does your body feel to you, does it feel like it needs to be cleaned out? That simple question about how you feel can help you ascertain if you have enough cleansing food and drink. Life is broad and varied, and naturally you want to have food that tastes great and is fun. But be sure to consider the entire context of your diet. You can certainly eat for fun but you need to eat for your health, vitality, and life first. This is the only life you have! Feed it well and make sure to have a little fun and excitement too.

The applied principle for this step is to add food and drink that help to clean and cleanse your system.

CHAPTER 11

EAT FOODS THAT AID DIGESTION

Being aware of how you feel, how and when you go to the bathroom, and observing when you experience indigestion can be essential in learning what foods are helping you and building you up and what foods are making things worse for you or are breaking down your system.

Put more clinically, you'll be able to tell which foods stimulate your ability to break things down, absorb nutrients, and eliminate waste. And which ones cause your digestion to be impeded, damage your ability to absorb resources, or slow down efficient and appropriate elimination of waste and by-products.

Years ago, I worked with a client who couldn't get rid of his backache or get the tension to subside. I knew he had seen his physician and was in generally good health. I finally asked him if his bowels were regular and he said, "Oh yeah, I go every seven days like clockwork." I'm guessing most of you already know that this is not enough, but some people don't really know what would be considered "normal." For this client, after all, weekly bowel movements were "normal." I sent him back to his physician and they did some emergency work to get his intestines functioning.

Our digestive system works by breaking things down, absorbing the nutrients, and then eliminating the waste. If you're having problems with any one of these factors, you may develop health and vitality problems. Even if you eat the best food and drink the cleanest water in the world, you're facing a lot of potential problems with your health, weight, and energy levels if you are unable to break it down and absorb the nutrients efficiently. So we want to start paying attention to how our system functions in regard to these processes.

Some people can digest a rock coated with fiery devil sauce and they will have no indigestion. They will still get some nutrients from it, and they will continue to eliminate as regularly as a train schedule (and more than once a week). Other people have to be very conscious of what they eat, when they eat, and how they eat, and these people can still have problems, even with the best food and drink.

In almost all cases, I think this can be improved or completely healed with the right interventions and by working with the right medical professionals. But it's also important to take ownership of your relationship to food and your body and get a baseline for where you are now. From there, you can improve.

Work with medical professionals

Talk to your doctor to see if you have medical problems. But then do your own research on food and how it affects humans. Then, think about how you might use it to benefit yourself and your life. For decades, I was told I just had a genetic problem and so I should live on acid blockers and diarrhea medications but that answer was insufficient for me. Ultimately, it turned out to be wrong.

It took an enormous amount of research and playing with variables to make a difference for myself. I had to try new doctors and alternative health models until I found the answers I needed. Once I learned I had infections interfering with every aspect of my digestion, I worked with my doctor to kill them. I was able to make incredible improvements. I coupled that with using what I learned about ancient and alternative health practices and working with an acupuncturist to improve even further. These methods also helped me keep going when I was in incredible pain and unable to digest much.

Unless you've been forced to pay attention to your digestive system because you have a condition with chronic digestion problems, you may not be too aware of how your digestive system works for you. The following is a short list of questions to help you gauge how your digestion functions. It's just a primer, really, to get you started. Please take additional notes about whatever is working well to help you get your mind around the concept. It can be quite helpful to revisit your answers as you develop your understanding of this important issue. You might be surprised how well you can attend to your digestion if you listen to your body with sensitivity and attention.

As a general rule, if you don't have pain when you eat, are pooping most days, aren't regularly experiencing diarrhea or constipation, don't have burning in your gut or throat, and aren't burping often, your digestion is probably in the ballpark of healthy. You can still fine tune it quite a bit (some experts say you should poop after each meal). There are also little triggers that can indicate problems with digestion, such as acid reflux, which can show itself in coughing, often when you lie down.

Take your time to work through these questions.

- How well would you say your digestion works, generally speaking?
  - Does your digestion seem to work well? Does it feel like your body easily breaks things down? If you have never had to think about it, you might have excellent digestion.
  - Do you have pain after you eat, or do you feel really sluggish after a meal?

- How much of the food you eat is whole versus processed? Half? More than half? Less than?

- Do you cook? Learning to cook (or expanding your techniques and knowledge, if you already do) can help. Some cooking styles are very helpful in releasing elements in the food to help digestion, and you might find other ways of preparing food that make it more difficult for you. Over-cooked, dry food can be tough to break down, for example.

- Do you experience pain when you eat? This is a fairly sure sign that something isn't quite right. (If you have always had pain you might think it is more normal than it actually is. Many people with chronic illnesses don't realize that what they're going through isn't normal.)

- Do some foods constipate you? You might need a journal to catch this. If something is a regular part of your food regimen, it may be hard to spot it without some way to track things or working with an elimination-type diet.

- Do some foods help your digestion? The acids in certain foods, like lemons and limes, can help you to break down food. Certain combinations of food can help your system do well, while others might be a no-no. The right spices can also help. For some people, those might be the "hot" spices but it could also be spices like turmeric, coriander, or fennel.

- Do some foods help you to eliminate? To be specific, some food and drink will help you poop and others will stop you up like rush-hour traffic. This is worth really playing with because it can be very individualized and certain combinations can have a large effect.

- Do you eat food with probiotics? It's easy to neglect the probiotics in our food and just take supplements. It can be helpful to add probiotic-rich food into your diet with each meal. Kefir (a yogurt-like drink), Greek yogurt, raw sauerkraut (you can make it at home or buy it at a health food store), raw kimchee, and miso are all good choices.

- Do you eat food with prebiotics? These are compounds in foods that help the growth of beneficial bacteria in the gastrointestinal tract. Raw garlic, onions, bananas, and dandelion greens are good sources. (On a side note, almost all of these are quite tough on my own digestion, so please be careful with all suggestions and test them for yourself carefully. Some things won't work for you; we all have our unique and individual characteristics, which is truly wonderful, so be kind enough to yourself to eat in the way that serves you best.)

Another thing to consider is how much your emotions, mental state, and activities affect your capacity for digestion. This is easy to see in times of massive, immediate stress. What happens to your body as you're eating when your boss calls to threaten your job? Or your significant other is intent on picking a fight? How much stress is needed to create a negative impact on your digestive system?

Let's take something common, like eating while watching the news. What do you think your digestion is doing while you are hearing stories of politics, rape, murder, and genocide? When you are watching that, some part of you is stressed. That's not going to help your digestive function. You are unconsciously activating the sympathetic nervous branch of your autonomic nervous system. When this system is working, your body is prioritizing activities like running and fighting over digestion.

Take some time for yourself

Give yourself a quiet, safe, relaxing, and enjoyable space and time to eat. Make your body amenable to digestion and healing. At some point you want to take yourself out of the "stress battlefield" and let things rebuild, heal, and grow. Look at something beautiful and uplifting, have a pleasant conversation with friends or family, watch a beautiful sunset, and observe and enjoy your food. Those little things can make a large change in your ability to digest, absorb, and eliminate because you aren't working at cross-purposes with yourself.

These are just a few easy-to-implement methods for changing your responses to our increasingly busy, stressful, and active lives. There is so much more to say on this topic and so much more to teach about how to work with our minds, emotions, and bodies to live healthier, calmer, more sustainable, and more directly controllable lives in regard to our stress.

The applied principle for this step is to eat foods that help digestion and eat in such a way that your body can focus on digestion.

CHAPTER 12

EAT A BROAD VARIETY

O ur bodies need and use a large variety of substances in order to run well. Consider the list of vitamins and minerals in a multivitamin. We want our diet to include as many of the nutrients in appropriate proportions as we can reasonably achieve. One way to increase our chances of getting what we need is through eating a broad variety of foods, as well as trying to get as much variety of colors in our veggies and fruit.

Sadly, gummy bears and Skittles don't count—we're aiming to eat a different kind of rainbow. I read some useful ancient advice when I was a teenager about trying to get five colors of food in each meal: You might have green beans, white rice, red peppers, carrots, and eggplant. This can be difficult to do all the time, but it makes a good point and is a good standard to strive for. More variety in your food gives you more access to what you need as fuel for your body, and this will allow you to live life more closely to the way you want.

It would be problematic to give very definite rules for how much of these you should include in your diet at any given time. In general, work on including a few into your diet daily. For most people, five to seven might be a good target. There's a lot of room for variation depending on what works best for your particular genetics and digestion. For some people, adding too many variations and combinations can upset digestion. For example, a popular Chinese dish called Buddha's Delight has a rich mix of veggies in a light sauce. For some, this mix of veggies is taxing on digestion. For others, it's the perfect way to incorporate a wide variety of veggies in one meal. You need to pay attention to how this affects you. You may need to limit yourself to two or three in a meal, and you might find certain combinations are helpful while others make you feel tired or sluggish.

For people who have real trouble with digestion, you might try finely blending a few veggies and putting them into bone broth, miso soup, or a veggie broth. Be careful with a tomato-based soup; for some people the nightshade family of flowering plants can be troublesome. That family also includes eggplant, bell and chili peppers, potatoes, and interestingly, tobacco.

A wealth of variety

There are many vegetables, fruits, nuts, seeds, mushrooms, greens, spices, meats, and fish to choose from. It can be fun and useful to take a little safari through all the options that you can find, and learn how people traditionally prepare them. People around the world have been preparing food in all kinds of interesting and appetizing ways for thousands of years. Some you will love and some won't suit your taste very well. But this is a great way to start to add spice to your life and nutrients to your diet. It's easy to stay with what you know, what's easy, and what your family has always eaten, but there are lots of options out there to expand your palate and your experience of life. Once you've expanded your world, you can build a bigger, more expansive diet of foods you like and foods that build your health, vitality, and life.

In particular, try to add more vegetables. Look at diets from around the world that are famous for their health-building qualities and for creating cultures of long life, like the Okinawan diet. Try new ways of preparing food and adding flavors you haven't used very often. It could be a real adventure into new parts of the world and into new parts of yourself. Spices can be helpful in this endeavor and remember: Spices don't have to be "hot." There are a wide variety of spices to engage your senses, aid in digestion, and change the overall tone of food. Spices can keep things interesting for you. You could take a trip around the world through spices and different methods of preparing food. There are so many flavors to try, colors to add, and health benefits to reap, you might be pleasantly surprised. Learning to cook well can be an art form and it can improve your relationship with food.

Learning to cook can transform food from a boring, automatic, chemical "fix" into an experience to enjoy and share with people you care about. It can be a wonderful way to lift yourself out of the dumps and add to your life and enjoyment of life. You can also use your daily life with food as a means to travel and explore the world and see and relate to new cultures. Today, you could explore the cuisine of Japan and learn about the ways they have traditionally viewed food. Tomorrow, you could experience the food art of Ethiopia or Peru. You probably won't like everything. No worries! Part of what you are doing is expanding yourself and your life. And you can do it without having to leave your city or region!

Experience life

You might open a door in yourself that you may not have opened any other way. For example, on one of my trips to Japan I got to experience eating natto, which is made from fermented soy beans.

It has a particular smell and texture that is hard to find in many other foods, especially in North American cuisine. At first, the smell hit me like an olfactory brick but now I really enjoy it. I don't eat it often but it opened my eyes to new foods, textures, and the health benefits of foods outside my experience. Now I'm a bit more on the adventurous side, but you don't have to go that far if you don't want to. There are plenty of options out there. When you eat out, try asking the waitstaff about the food you ordered and how it's prepared, especially if you're eating food from other cultures, like India or Vietnam. Indian food is known for its sophisticated and complex use of spices, so you can learn a lot by talking to your server and asking questions. This can help you get a feel for and understanding about foods and how they are prepared. With this kind of exploration, you can open your eyes and stomach to a new world, and from these experiences you can build a daily diet that suits your needs, your health, and your individual sense of adventure and novelty. Now you have a base from which to build your food knowledge.

These questions will help you find ways to incorporate some new and unusual veggies into your diet:

- How can you add some fresh veggies to one of your meals today? Adding one counts!

- Make a list of vegetables you've never tried. The next time you are shopping, take your time in the produce section and note the ones you've never picked up, and add them to this list.

- For each vegetable you haven't tried, can you find one way it is traditionally prepared?

- Can you find a simple, new-to-you recipe that you can try today or on your next day off? It's okay if you end up disliking it. A consistent effort will broaden your horizons until you find things that you do like.

If you don't know how to cook, this would be a good time to learn a few recipes. Perhaps, you have a friend who wants to learn to cook or expand his or her cooking horizons. Practice together and share a meal.

Start simple and with something tasty that you like and build from there. It's easier than ever to get instructions on how to cook. There are many channels on YouTube and an abundance of books out there to help you get started. You could even take a class at a community college or cooking school. Some grocery stores even offer cooking classes!

Having people around you who are also learning to cook, or who love to cook, can be helpful as a means to get going. It might also be useful and fun to try new ethnic cuisines the next time you eat out. Even if you eat a particular kind of ethnic food with some regularity, like Thai or Chinese, challenge yourself to try a new dish or two next time. It doesn't need to be super racy, just something new. Have some fun, go on an adventure, and spice up your life!

Remember: This is all a grand experiment about what works best for you. I provide a few directions and recommendations, but it's up to you to play with things while being present and "in" your body as much as possible. Try to distill out the principle and then make it work well for you.

The applied principle for this step is eat a variety of foods that can help you get the nutrition that you need.

CHAPTER 13

LEAVE SOME SPACE TO DIGEST

Digestion works best when you leave enough room for your stomach and intestines to do their jobs. For them to work effectively, there needs to be enough room for your stomach acid to penetrate the food so it can be broken down. The tissues need enough space to efficiently move the food down your digestive tract.

These days, we often eat until we need to be rolled home after almost every meal. We eat so quickly our body doesn't have time to send the signal of satiety before we finish our five cheeseburgers. Many of our food habits are completely out of line for what we want most in our lives and for our health. We need to take stock of this situation. A good measure is to shoot for something around 70 percent full, including whatever you are drinking. Don't tax your system by filling up too much.

In order to change this tendency, it can be helpful to consider these next questions.

- Why do people eat way past the point they should stop?
  - With kindness, ask yourself now, why do you do this? When do you do this?

- Why do some people barely eat enough to sustain themselves?
  - If you do, ask yourself, with compassion, why?

Here are some basic reasons to consider.

People don't pay attention to what they eat. They're busy or rushed. They grab whatever's quick and easy from the fridge. Others aren't getting the nutrients they need from the food they do eat so their bodies urge them to eat more. This happens often when eating. Some folks eat more than their share because it's the only pleasure they get. They can't afford any luxuries because they're focused on making ends meet. Food is the only reward they seem to get these days.

Still others were raised to finish everything on their plate. They don't want any of it to go to waste, especially when "there are starving people out there."

No doubt you could add many more reasons to this list, but find your own reasons and put some attention on your ways of doing things and your habits. There's an interesting life lesson here: You can only use so much at one time. More is not always better, and in fact you almost always begin to damage something when you go too far. How do you know when enough is enough? How do you know when you have the perfect amount? Can you recognize when you need to stop?

Take the time to practice

Practice this skill of learning when to stop in every area of life. Put your attention on when you have too little or too much of something in your life. Too little and too much sleep are bad for your health. Too little or too much weight-lifting can damage your vitality. It may seem that this is going off the topic of food, but the same tendency found in your food habits can easily exist in other areas of your life. Working on the overall tendency can be valuable in changing that propensity with food. Stay present and know when you got the most out of what you are doing in regard to what you want to accomplish.

The questions below are meant to help you change your perspective and get a little distance from yourself. This approach will help you understand why you have a tendency to overdo, underdo, or hold yourself back. Take a few minutes and write down the answers to these questions. You might find them applicable to many aspects of your life. Be clear with yourself but also be kind. Being judgmental and attacking yourself can exaggerate the behaviors you use as coping mechanisms, and it will always take you out of being here and in this moment. Remember: the only place you can work is here and now.

Before we begin, are you a person who generally goes to extremes or do you stay near complacency? What does it get you? You learned so much of this when you were young, and you might think these tendencies are just who you are. Seeing clearly is the first step to getting closer to a sustainable, healthy middle path.

These questions might be a little bit difficult, so be honest with yourself but do so with kindness:

- Generally speaking, do you believe more is always better? Do you think this is broadly true or simply true for you?

- When was the last time you overdid something good? Why did you overdo?

CHAPTER 14

PULL VITALITY OUT OF FOOD

D o you consciously realize and understand that you are getting energy for your life from your food? You probably know this on an abstract level, but what would you change if you considered that the energy used to write your book, play with your kids, fight cancer, study for school, work out, love your spouse, play with your dogs, go on vacation, feel joy, feel happiness, and to just be you comes in a major way from the food you eat? With that realization consciously observed, would you change what you choose to eat? If you could consciously add that understanding to your daily life, what would change?

Do you know in a visceral way that a salad with grilled chicken gives you more sustainable health and vitality than a candy bar with two beers? Do you know you are playing with your health and vitality when you eat junk food regularly? Of course, this is a much bigger conversation than just counting calories; it goes into how food affects your metabolism, your hormones, and many of the processes affecting how your body creates the energy that you need. Don't we all want to be more vital in order to chase our dreams and our dream life?

It can be helpful to keep a journal in which you record your energy levels and the food you eat. Use it to track what gives you the most resources (energy, vitality, clarity of thought, emotional stability) when you eat it. It doesn't matter if you write your journal on paper or on your phone, computer, or iPad. Whatever works, use that. You can change your method anytime you feel like it—just break the inertia right now.

Alongside of writing down what you eat, keep track of how you feel emotionally, mentally, physically, socially, and internally.

This shouldn't take more than a few minutes to set up and then about one minute each time you eat and before you go to bed. It doesn't need to look good, it doesn't need to make sense to anyone but you, and it doesn't need to please your third-grade teacher or your mom. It just has to work for you, here and now. Five minutes of doing something could help you begin to change your life. Get the ball moving. Do it now.

How does food affect you?

Over time you can begin to see how foods affect you. Does the food you eat give you more with which to run your life or does it make life more difficult? If you eat pizza and ice cream three days in a row, how does that affect your daily routine? Does it make life difficult or does it make it easy? Over the week, if you eat more whole, nutritious foods that are well-prepared, does that give you more joie de vivre for the weekend when you get to take your kids to the pool or go see that concert?

As I have often said in this book, this is your life. Most people have had this understanding knocked out of them, and that's why I'm trying to knock it back into you. These questions are fundamental to recovering some of what has been lost in our socialization as we grew up. Be serious about the answers, but make the process enjoyable and kind of fun. This should be a natural process of self-discovery and making it difficult will block the process.

- What could you do if you had 20 percent more energetic resources available in how you perceive and felt available energy for the day and for your life? Think about your dreams and how you want to live your life: what could you do with that 20 percent?
  - What would you be able to accomplish?
  - What would you be able to see?
  - What dreams would you be able to realize?

- Have you become consciously aware of how food feeds you? Not just in a vague way but in a concrete way? If not, this is your chance.

- Have you noticed that how you feel emotionally is connected to the amount of energy you feel in your life and vice versa? Can you think of two or three specific examples?

- Have you eaten some foods that don't agree with you and then noticed that you felt irritable and grumpy? Which foods have this effect on you?

- When you've had periods of eating meals that nourish, have you noticed the effect? Is your mood more stable? Can you be enthusiastic without really having to work at it? Connecting the dots and bringing these relationships into conscious awareness is an important step.

One of the reasons many people overeat or under eat is that they feel no purpose in their daily life. If you have purpose coming from inside, it can help you fill the hole now being filled by food.

This will give you a strong source of vitality, which is another form of food. "Purpose food," if you like.

Of course, there are many factors contributing to how much energy you feel. How much and how well you sleep and illness are major players as well, but changing how you see food, and becoming aware of its influence on your vitality, could potentially change the entire pattern of your life. You might just have the energy to finish your degree, to sculpt the new body you dream of, to play with your kids with enthusiasm, to create the life of your dreams. What would that be worth to you? What would you be willing to trade for that?

Where is your attention?

Paying attention to what you eat, *while* you eat, and concurrently paying attention to your body and your feelings, is one way to help you pull vitality out of your food. You will gain an understanding of what food is bringing to your body and what you feel about that food. You will learn if it is having a positive or negative impact on your body.

This might take some time and practice to master. It's actually quite meditative and calming, once you get the hang of it. It can make a large impact on the vitality you feel now and going forward into the future. It's also a wonderful way to begin building a stronger, more conscious mind-body connection. It will add to the currency of life available for your day, especially if you practice it long-term, which is especially useful if you are struggling with chronic health issues.

Would it be worth changing how you see food and your diet to get more vitality and energy?

The applied principle for this step is to eat foods and in such a way that you feel more vital.

CHAPTER 15

WHAT INFORMATION ARE YOU TAKING IN?

F ood is information, and it is communicating with your system. What is this food instructing your system to do? What does broccoli teach that nutrient-empty, sugary desserts do not? Ultimately, we are telling our body something important by what we eat, do, think, and feel, so if we can become conscious of this principle about food, we can slowly change how we choose what to eat. Changing how we relate to food on a deep level, consciously allows us to actually begin to view it differently. In this chapter, we will think about the information food sends to our body, mind, and emotions.

Let's look at food as a "program" we are installing into our computer. What are we programming our body, mind, and emotions to do with each meal? What is this food providing or delivering in its physical coding, which here takes the form of vitamins, fats, proteins, amino acids, minerals, and genetic material? How does it emotionally and mentally deliver information to you either consciously or unconsciously?

Are we programming health, vitality, fitness, clarity, stability, and cheerfulness? Or are we programming in "viruses" that will undermine our health, vitality, and peace of mind?

Again, I am not saying to never eat food that is bad for you but rather to consider what this food (especially in excess) teaches your system to do. What is the right amount for you and your needs? Where does your food lead you? Meals are a way to code for your health, vitality, fitness, emotional and mental health, and the life of your dreams, as well as having fun and enjoyment in the moment.

To provide a specific example: what does that pork chop give you nutritionally, and how does it make you feel?

Traditional philosophies and medicines all over the world point to a vital principle which is found in food among other places. Chinese call it qi, Japanese call it ki, and Indians call it prana. This energetic vital principle is found to a greater or lesser degree in the food you eat and how you have prepared it. The more natural the food you eat, the more of this energy you can "upload" from your food. Well-prepared broccoli has more qi than a heavily processed, two-year-old, chemically preserved protein bar. Some people consider such notions old-fashioned, but I urge you to play with this concept in your food during your daily diet. (By the way, which has been more heavily advertised to you: the two-year-old, processed protein bar or the newly grown organic broccoli? Why do you think that is?)

The way food is prepared will have a large impact on the information we take from it. We want food prepared in the way that gives us the most out of it, and we also want it to taste good. There are many ways to prepare food to make it more available to you and to make it more delicious.

Have fun with this! When you are planning a meal, think about balancing these two aspects of the food you'll prepare.

The applied principle for this step is to consider what the food you eat and what you drink are teaching your system by what information that food has in it.

CHAPTER 16

WHAT WILL YOU DO WITH THE ENERGY?

Food is power, so what do you do with the energy you're getting from your meals? Are you eating a 3,000-calorie meal to watch a full series of Netflix today? Are you fueling up to run a marathon, or laying down stores for the snowy season? Will you be lecturing to a group of 30 adults, or teaching a class of wild kindergartners? Are you loading for some heavy deadlifts and squats, or are you cutting back to get ready for a fitness competition? Are you going to work 12 hours today, or will you spend most of the day snuggled up and watching rom-coms?

Considering which foods to eat to suit your life and lifestyle could become a potent way to decide what and when to eat. Loading up on carbohydrates before a day sitting in front of the TV might not be the best method for you to accomplish your long-term goals, but carbo-loading might be useful before your strenuous endurance event. Eating a heavy farmer's breakfast might be useful if you are spending 12 hours in the field but might wreak havoc on your metabolism if you're an accountant who also snacks all day.

When you begin to plan, control, and create your life consciously, you can expect some life changes. So often people languish behind a series of unexamined habits and simply follow what they were taught and what was modeled. But whose life is this?

What kind of life do you want to have? What does that look like? Once you're clear about that, you can build a diet and lifestyle that leads to it. Don't forget: You are feeding your life with what you eat. It doesn't need to be perfect; it just needs to head in the direction you want to go over time. You don't have to live on chicken breast and broccoli, but if you want to be fit and healthy you can't live mostly on sugary snacks, soda, and blind anger.

We want to make food serve us in our lives rather than have us be the lapdog of our food and our transient desires. I hope I said that emphatically and clearly enough. Do you want to be at the mercy of your desires for food? Would you rather be the monarch of your life and your experience of it?

Hopefully, thinking about that pissed you off a little bit. Hopefully, it woke you up a little. Who or what is in control of you? Do you want to control your life and yourself?

There is a positive way out of this dilemma. This set of questions can help you apply this principle and develop a new way of seeing the relationship between the food you eat and the desired effect on your situation today.

Consider the day ahead:

- What kind of day will you have today? What's on your schedule?
  - Do you need to be mentally sharp today, or can you be groggy (sometimes you have the time to be a little groggy)?

- How do you need or want to feel?
- Do you need to think clearly and concisely for a specific purpose?

- Is today a cheat day? If it is, did you earn it appropriately?

- What exercises will you do today to help motivate your metabolism?

- What do you want to create with the energy and resources from your food?

- Are you planning to avoid foods that make you feel dull, drowsy, and emotional?

Consider the day you just completed:

- Did you plan your day to build toward the life you want? How do you need to eat to support that?

- If your day was very active, did you get enough food for the day?

- If your day was fairly inactive, did you make a healthy, calorie-appropriate meal plan for the day?

- If you ate emotionally, did you give yourself a little healthier option to create a limit for yourself? (By nature, emotional eating isn't this conscious, but if you play with this method for a while it will become more conscious for you.)

Finally, ask yourself these questions from a broader perspective:

- Do you know what times of day you eat that can make you groggy?

- What are you trying to build?

- Do you control your food by the life you want to lead, or does the food you eat control you and your life?

In a sense, this is an easy principle to apply once you understand the need for it. Excess resources get turned into storage. A little storage is okay but a lot begins to overwhelm the system.

The applied principle for this step is to eat the right amount of food for the expenditure of energy you will have during the day.

CHAPTER 17

MORE EMOTIONALLY IN CONTROL AND MORE LIKE YOURSELF

Ultimately, don't we all want to have some control over our inner life and our emotions? Many small, daily actions have a profound effect on how we feel emotionally. Sleep, for example, has a fairly large effect on our mood. Mindset is an important influence, as well. What, why, when, how, where, and with whom we eat all contribute to our emotional state.

This principle can call attention to how food affects emotions, and what direction to go in order to get the most out of the relationship between food and our emotions.

Eat foods that make you feel more emotionally in control and help you feel more like yourself. Consider how this food you are about to eat will affect you emotionally, and how it will affect how you feel about yourself and life. For example, will it produce a huge high with a crashing low? Or will it be so boring and bland that you lose some interest in life? Maybe it will be interesting and leave you feeling capable and good about yourself. It may be easy to miss the value in this, but please take a minute to think this through. Why do people spend so much money, time, and effort on food? Is it because they are worried about what vitamins they will get from the food, or is it because it changes their emotional state?

We use food and the dining experience to alter how we feel. In many ways, our mood might be the single biggest reason why people eat foods that they know aren't that good for their health! Our choices can produce a powerful change to our inner emotional state. This can be a useful tool in a moment, but it comes with a heavy cost (or benefit!) when used regularly over a long period of time.

Become consciously aware of how your food changes your state as a whole over time. So rather than just considering its impact on your state right now, think about how it will make you feel this week or this month. How long does the emotional charge you get from the piece of cake last? How do you feel when that charge ends? Eating the wrong foods can easily become an emotional roller coaster without end, and it can be very difficult to find a time to get off the wild ups and downs. But keen consciousness and observation of how food affects you emotionally can help you to identify a stable place to make a change.

Eat foods that help you feel more in control emotionally and help you feel the most like who you are authentically. This will take some real playing with if you are stuck on that up and down roller coaster of using foods to give you an easy emotional "hit" of pleasure. This will also take some mindful exploration, especially if you have chronic health problems.

Consider this from a longer-term perspective: It can affect your entire life. There is a very useful middle path between eating anything and everything that brings good feelings now, and eating only food that benefits your health and vitality but brings no emotional pleasure or positive change in state. In fact, many people feel great resentment when they have to eat foods they dislike with nothing pleasurable to offset that moment's emotional state.

The key

Eat foods that bring you longer-term emotional benefits as well as health and vitality. This will need to be an artistic blending of foods, and the process and discovery can be fun! However, this can take some time because there are some foods that will act like an emotional bomb.

Sometimes this takes the form of a memory. You might really enjoy greasy tacos because they remind you of a birthday you loved or that you were eating them the first time you fell in love. More immediately, eating half a cake with a carton of ice cream is massively powerful in changing your state for a little while but then drops you like a sack of bricks. When you are in that state you'll be craving a high (or enough energy) to get you back off the ground. That leaves you susceptible and driven to find another emotional bomb.

Proportioning your food and regulating the timing lets you learn to eat in a way that leaves you emotionally in control and helps you be yourself. Eating half a piece of cake with a scoop of ice cream might let you have some fun without dropping you so far down emotionally. Eating a well-balanced meal (determined by how it makes you function) before you eat the cake might help you stay emotionally even while also giving you a little bit of lifted emotional state.

Going to extremes is the enemy here; you can schedule a short food explosion of tastiness or set aside a useful period of healing and eating in as disciplined a way as possible. Both should be consciously planned and developed in the overall context of your food, health, and life needs. The food you eat should serve this principle: what helps you feel in control emotionally and helps you feel like your best self?

Another thing to consider is that if you are constantly eating while in a state of stress, your body will struggle to absorb the nutrients needed to process the food well since it's primed for other actions. Eating while driving and having a fight with your spouse at rush hour, for instance, is almost certainly going to make things difficult for your digestion, absorption, and elimination. Your body will begin to be starved of what it needs and that is bound to have an effect on its ability to produce what you need to function well—and that will have an effect on your mood and your emotions.

Eating well is more than just a useful way to control your waistline. It also has profound effects on your emotional state. Wouldn't it be life-changing to be healthy enough to have access to whatever emotions are useful and needed at the time we require them? Wouldn't it be useful to develop conscious control over ourselves so we can have the inner environment that is generally the way we want it? No one wants to be stuck in a state of down, tired, and grumpy. No one wants to be so exhausted they are scared (or unable) to chase their dreams. Whatever you take into your inner world will have an effect on your emotions. Remember, food directly affects your chemistry.

Learning to eat in order to build more emotional possibilities can be liberating. It's a subtle change at first, but if you play with building your diet in an intelligent, methodical, and organized way, you can begin to create change in your life. Look for the implications of this. It includes everything you take into your inner world, including TV, movies, music, and even interactions with friends.

In our culture we tend to treat emotions as if they are us, like they're something we can't control or like they're something to be beaten down and ignored. None of these ways of working with emotions will lead you very far in the search for health, vitality, or inner wealth. Everything we do, think, or feel has a large impact on our emotional landscape.

One of the coolest ways to start changing your emotional environment is to play with food in such a way that it helps your emotional state to become what you want it to be.

And this leads us into the way food also has a relationship with how we think.

The applied principle for this step is to eat in such a way that you feel more emotionally in control and like yourself.

CHAPTER 18

IN ORDER TO THINK CLEARLY, SHARPLY, AND CONCISELY

In the previous chapter, we scratched the surface of the two-way relationship between food and our emotions. In this chapter, we'll explore how food can affect our thoughts and thought processes. Our brains are built and fueled by what we eat. Blood sugar levels, for example, have an interesting impact on how well our brains function.

Have you noticed how much your diet can affect the way you think, process information, apply yourself on tests, function in meetings, or make intelligent, well thought-out decisions? Have you ever had a huge meal with a large dessert afterwards and noticed you were a bit slow, muddled, or simply unable to connect the dots as quickly as you might normally? Have you had the experience of mind fog after the wrong meal at the wrong time?

Take some time over the next few weeks to observe how you function while asking yourself these questions. Use your food journal for more accurate answers:

- What foods help my mind to work quickly and sharply?

- What foods bring me down into a mind fog or sluggish and sloppy thinking?

Your brain is built from and runs on food. It burns resources mined from your food; it isn't generating something out of nothing. Eating the right diet can help you maximize your mind's ability to function. The better your mind functions, the better the chance you'll make purposeful, proper judgments and decisions. This won't guarantee you make the right decisions for you and your life because your operating premises and the motivations that drive you may be off but that is a discussion for another time. For now, try to figure out what foods help you think clearly and what foods make you feel slow, confused, and groggy. Then move your diet in the direction of foods that support clear thinking. It is very important to note that if you radically change your diet to one that is much healthier for you, you might struggle to think sharply and to feel emotionally up for a while. When you change your diet, it can create a kind of shock to the system. Stick with it! If you can gently push through this phase, you will come out the other side in a better place than you are now.

If it becomes difficult, you may want to seek the advice of a health professional who specializes in nutrition and diet. If you find yourself struggling a great deal emotionally or mentally, don't hesitate to get the help of a therapist, counselor, or another professional who's trained and qualified to help you. This is a very important part of your life, so use any available source to help you move in the direction of the greatest health, vitality, life, and your dreams.

Remember that this is a rather large transition and change you're making to your life. Someone once told me that they didn't want to work on their health because they didn't want to live a long life. That statement suggested to me this person didn't feel very well and felt that life was beating them down pretty hard. Feeling healthy, vital, strong, and clear might change such a perspective, and eating properly can help move you fundamentally in that direction.

The effects of food and diet on your mind are quite powerful, so take a little time to explore the effects of your diet to see what gives you the clearest, most stable and energized way of thinking. You might focus on this in your journal if it seems like a critical issue for your life. It takes some observation and personal exploration. It isn't as simple as just eating a bunch of blueberries because they have antioxidants in them or taking gingko biloba because it has been shown to help people think clearly. They might help you but this is a bigger picture. Everything fits together to make a complete puzzle. A bowl of blueberries probably won't offset something that makes you feel fuzzy-headed. Find what makes you fuzzy-headed and be decisive enough to boot it out of your diet.

A few things to specifically consider are sugars, potential food allergies, flavor enhancers, food coloring, timing of meals, hydration, fasting, size of meals, how fast you eat, and food combinations. If mental clarity is an issue for you, track these in your food journal too. All these factors affect people differently and will affect their thinking processes differently. Our bodies are connected to our brains, and this is an important consideration when you are trying to change your diet, vitality, health, and enjoyment of your time and your life.

Take care of your stomach because it will help you take care of your mind.

The applied principle for this step is to eat in such a way that you feel mentally capable.

CHAPTER 19

BE GRATEFUL FOR
THE FOOD YOU EAT

Finally, we come to the principle of gratitude itself as a form of food. Genuinely feeling thankful for the food we eat is a wonderful and useful way to make a large change in your relationship to food as a whole. It helps trigger a feeling of satiety. It can help shut down the feeling of needing more to be full. When you begin to consciously remember and feel that you are fortunate to have what you have and to eat what you are eating, the feelings of needing more and more begin to cave in on themselves. It is a lovely way to begin to do away with the emotional need to keep trying to fill yourself up.

It's important to clarify here that I'm talking about actually feeling real gratitude, feeling thankful for what you have. This is not about shame or guilt. It can be easy to confuse these feelings because many of us were raised to feel guilty and ashamed for what we have. It can be easy to slide into feeling horrible about yourself because you have something rather than taking a positive approach and being genuinely grateful for what is in your life.

For the purpose of this specific discussion about food, feeling bad about yourself is likely to aggravate the behaviors you want to eliminate, whereas feeling thankful is a strongly positive state and will fill you up inside in a different way. That can help reduce the emotional need for binging to feel good about yourself and life.

Gratitude helps you feed the deeper parts of you. In many ways it's like taking the time to prepare a healthy and nutritious meal for your emotions and mind. Consider: With what emotions are you feeding yourself? What emotions feed and nourish you, and which ones make you ravenous for more or are damaging to your long-term health? Do general feelings of negativity leave you feeling fulfilled, or does filling yourself with enthusiasm or love fill a part of you that can't be filled any other way?

It's easy to eat in order to fill an emotional hole. Perhaps, we have all done it. You begin to feel empty inside, and in an attempt to fill that inner lack, food is an easily available substitute for something that's harder to find, or perhaps intangible. Creating an "emotional diet" is very helpful, and gratitude is the perfect place to start.

Telling yourself that you appreciate what you have eaten towards the end of the meal is a great way to begin applying this principle. At first you can say it to yourself, or even out loud, but concentrate on feeling it instead of mindlessly saying it. Once you feel it a little bit, try to amplify the feeling. If you do this regularly it will pick up some momentum in your life and with your diet.

Use this in your daily life

Naturally, you don't need to wait until you are eating to feed yourself with gratitude. You can use this principle at any time, and it is useful

CHAPTER 20

HOW TO USE THE NLM FOOD LADDER

For those of you who want the goods right now

You can take any one of these principles and make them work a hundred different ways. The principles need to serve you and your needs, not the other way around.

That said, this ladder approach is useful for learning to create a change through the use of a set of principles. It creates a big enough shock to the system that encourages it to build bigger and longer-lasting change. There are stacking principles within the NLM, but you might find yourself gravitating towards certain ideas at certain times. Honor that feeling if it happens. This chapter works whether you're the type who skips to the end of the book to get directly to the short and sweet description of how this works or if you're one of those who have read the book and want a short synopsis to quickly refresh your memory.

Here is the essence of the food ladder.

This is a method to apply at each meal. Use specific principles as you eat, in the form of steps considered at each meal, to apply changes in how you think, feel, sense, and act in regard to food.

I developed this system for myself, to make the changes I couldn't seem to create any other way. It requires you to build a series of habits, the first of which is to remember to go through this ladder each time you eat. Don't make it some sort of soul-crushing, painful ball and chain! Take your time, play with it, have some fun, and let the method work on you over time. If you do it right, you will begin to see changes that show up in your different thought processes, feelings toward yourself and food, and the way your body senses the food.

Embedded in this method are more than just principles about food. All the principles in this method will connect to other methods that make up the core of the Nytality Method; those will be available in future books and materials. Be careful about changing the basic formulas because later on you might miss the connections. So here we go...

Step One (Chapter 6): Say to yourself, "I eat to nourish myself and my life" before you eat or drink anything. You are programming this into your thinking process and habitual life so when you even think of food, this idea shows up. Use this idea over time and it will create a new gravity in the way you think. You'll begin to start with that idea rather than suddenly realizing you've eaten half a bag of chips and not knowing how you got there.

Step Two (Chapter 7): Get into your body and ask yourself, "Is there space needing to be filled?" Then feel and sense whether you really need food or drink or whether you're trying to fill a different need. We need to recover an almost childlike understanding of ourselves and reestablish an intimate relationship with our body and feelings. People often allow their mind and emotions to overrule their body in deciding whether or not to eat.

Step Three (Chapter 8): Is your metabolism stoked? Have you done any kind of activity to help your metabolism function well? Have you exercised, worked out, played, lifted, done isometrics, walked, run, trained, walked up the stairs, wrestled, or something of the sort? If you haven't, before you eat, try for some isometrics, or some squats, or take a quick walk.

Step Four (Chapter 9): Get the most out of your food. Is it well prepared? Does it offer more of what you need in the form of vitamins, minerals, fats, proteins, carbohydrates, and qi? Remember to chew appropriately as that allows you to get more out of the food. Take time to eat so your body can do its job well without making it extra difficult.

Step Five (Chapter 10): Eat and drink foods that clean and cleanse you. Help your body to function properly and efficiently by keeping it clean and cleansed. Your body is up to 60 percent water— more, if you are younger. Drinking clean, fresh water might be more useful than you think. Fiber is also important in this discussion. Have you eaten anything today to help keep your insides clean?

Step Six (Chapter 11): Eat foods that assist digestion, assimilation, elimination, and movement. Eat foods that help your ability to break down food, pick up as many of the food's nutrients as possible, and get rid of the waste effectively. Observe what helps and add some of that into your food daily. Low sugar yogurt or kefir, probiotic sauerkraut, foods with fiber, and eating a variety of veggies can be helpful.

Step Seven (Chapter 12): Eat a broad variety of nutrients, food groups, and colors within your veggies and fruit. At least once a day, try to add a reasonable variety of options to help your body get what it needs. Choose foods that are naturally colorful.

Step Eight (Chapter 13): Leave some space to digest your food and absorb what you drink. It's a wonderful habit to stop short of overdoing it. Have fun and go crazy on occasion, but don't try to do this until you have already set up the habit to stop before you are full.

Step Nine (Chapter 14): Pull vitality out of food. Remember while you eat that this food is fueling you. Get consciously into your body as you eat.

Step Ten (Chapter 15): What information are you taking in from your food and drink? The food you eat is providing resources and information your body uses to build and repair itself. Emotionally and mentally, it is also suggesting something to you about you. This will naturally be related to your belief system but some of it is straight chemistry and genetics.

Step Eleven (Chapter 16): What will you do with the energy (calories) from the food you're eating? Is the amount of food you are taking in proportional to the expenditure you will put out? Not every meal needs to be calorie dense. Consider your life today and tomorrow, what is the caloric output you will have?

Step Twelve (Chapter 17): Eat foods that leave you feeling more emotionally in control and more like yourself. How will this food affect you emotionally, and how will it affect the way you feel about yourself and your life?

Step Thirteen (Chapter 18): Eat the foods that help you think clearly, sharply, and concisely. Do the work to learn which foods make you sharper and which leave you in a fog.

Step Fourteen (Chapter 19): Be grateful for the food you eat and that you have enough to sustain you. Try to feel that way for at last five minutes.

A FAREWELL FOR THIS NEW JOURNEY

We have come to the end of our time together here. Now it is all about application and diligently working with the methods and making them work for you. Please use them any way you can to get them to work for YOU. Don't stop seeking answers and methods that will bring you the results and the life you desire.

When I was young I tripped over an ancient saying that has really stuck with me. I haven't been able to find it again, but I want to share this paraphrase: If you want to see that humans are crazy, look at how they live as if they will live forever but could die at any moment. It certainly is an interesting perspective and has the power to help you see the value of today and not waiting for someday to live the life that is in your heart. You might not get a chance because life is short.

Ultimately, your inner experience of life determines a major portion of how fulfilled you will feel and how life will seem and feel to you. The way you feed yourself has a large effect on how you experience life and how you build and manage your world. This is ultimately the crux of this method. How do you change your experience of life to get what you want out of it? How is it done consciously, successfully, and sustainably?

The ability to change things inside will also begin to change your external life. It seems like such a small idea: How I feed myself changes me and my life. But let's look at the ripple potential of that idea: If I feed myself well it will reverberate out into my environment and potentially have a positive impact on the people I care about. They may go to have a further impact on society. We are all nodes in a system, and it's hard to know how much of what we do on a personal level might affect the rest of the system.

Your relationship with food is a great place to start making a full life change. It's worth the time to explore yourself and the world through this process because it won't end with just food. The ideas can percolate through your life, health, and into your future.

I have many more principles and methods coming down the line. I invite you to keep in touch on my social media platforms and my website. I have a lot to share that has been deeply life-changing for me, and my hope is that it will do the same for you. I'll be relentlessly working to bring them to you, tools that can explode your experience of life into something more beautiful, tantalizing, magical, and fulfilling.

I'm developing bonus material to add to this information; send me your receipt from the purchase of this book and I'll forward those on to you as I finish them. I have some useful video content to help with digestion, exercise, and helping to keep yourself calm and energetic as you apply this material. This method is constantly expanding so please check back often.

Be relentless. Take good care of yourself because you matter. Don't let anyone convince you otherwise. Be quietly unstoppable.

Nytality.com
Instagram: Nyholmvitallifemethod
Twitter: @LifeNyholm

ADDENDUM

This last section is for those who haven't been able to make the changes they want or are generally struggling with applying the method. Even if you aren't, some of the material in this section may add to the process for you! You may feel like you know some of it already, but the reminder can be helpful in application or in finding a hole that you may have missed. I personally find these issues essential in changing one's relationship to food, but they aren't spelled out in the formal steps of the method.

How do you see yourself literally?

Ask yourself these questions with an open mind. They can help you uncover some subconscious programming about yourself. And remember: this is private, just for you.

The more honesty and clarity you can bring to the questions, the better.

- When you think about how your body looks, what do you see? This isn't about looking in the mirror, it's about your mental representation of your body, your ideas about how your body looks. Based on the image you hold, how would you describe it? Say it in words.
    - Is that description good, bad, or indifferent? Make this assessment for yourself. You're probably already aware of how our culture evaluates that body. Is that evaluation in your best interest? It is important to have

a viable standard. Ask yourself: Is the standard set forth by your culture based on your health and best interests? Or is it selling you something?

- Is that mental image what you actually look like?
  - Consider taking some pictures to compare. This might be frightening, off-putting, or just suck, but pictures are useful because you can look back at them later.

This isn't about trying meet societal expectations. It's about becoming aware of your body and the distortions we all seem to have regarding our physical form.

How can you make intelligent decisions about your health and vitality when you are working off broken or false information? Please keep in mind that this is for you and you alone. You don't have to prove anything to anyone if you don't want to. Whatever it is, it's okay to see. Once you see it, you can decide for yourself what you want to do about your body, health, vitality, and diet. There are almost always many options for making whatever changes you deem important.

You *aren't your body*. Please don't let the current and transitory state of it be the determining factor of your self-esteem. You are much greater than the shape of your body. Don't let anyone convince you of anything different. That also means you can make changes to your body. It is responsive to your actions, diet, thoughts, emotions, sleep, and exercise. It is also responsive to determined, disciplined effort.

Changing how you see your body is a huge determining factor in how you will exercise and diet. If you want to make big changes in your health and vitality, it will be helpful to begin working on the way you see yourself right now—specifically, the way you imagine yourself to be right now, the way you talk about yourself, and the way you feel about yourself.

Listen for the way you talk about yourself in regard to your body, your health, your vitality, and your strength. Listen carefully to your words and the tone of them, and experience all of that clearly. From there you can begin to change how you talk to and about yourself, how you imagine yourself, and how you feel about your body. That can help you change your diet, exercise, sleep, and perhaps most importantly, help you become okay with yourself.

Even better, it may help you begin to love yourself and your body. For many people, this one change could revolutionize their experience of life. How valuable would that be for you?

Difficulties giving up junk food, soda, desserts, and snacks

If you have grown up like many of us, you were raised with premade food designed to make you want to eat more. The bag of tricks includes additives, flavoring, irritants, sugar, corn syrup, cheap fats, carbonation, flavor enhancers, advertising, marketing, star power, and much more. This is very important to understand when you are changing your diet and, more importantly, your health. "They" have a serious financial motive to keeping you eating.

I'm not making sales departments, chemists, advertisers, and marketers the bad guys. It's just a fact of life: People are trying to sell you things. They sell more of what people buy. People buy more of what is made especially attractive, even if this isn't in their best interest. Ultimately, the responsibility lies with you. We are free to choose what we eat and what we don't eat. But if food is made to chemically entice you, then you'll need to anticipate that when you make significant changes in your diet.

I'll give you a personal example. Years ago, I was visiting my brother at his condo. I had just driven a few hours to get there and was hungry and sleepy from the road. Someone had left some French fries on the counter from a famous fast food joint, and I haphazardly ate one while chatting about the Broncos. I was genuinely disgusted by the cold, old French fry. It was slimy, smashed, and greasy. I sort of begrudgingly swallowed it to get the nasty taste out of my mouth. As I continued to talk with my brother and his friends about football and our plans for that night, all I could think about was eating another one of those nasty fries. My mouth was actually salivating. My eyes kept gravitating to them. And that one fry tasted like shit! But whatever they had put on it manipulated my chemistry and taste buds so I wanted almost desperately to have another one. This is something to think about. It disgusted me but I wanted more.

After a lifetime eating prepackaged food stuffed with flavor enhancers, a chicken breast, some cauliflower, and a glass of water is going to be boring. This isn't because chicken breast reasonably well-prepared doesn't taste good but because your taste buds were being directly manipulated before. This is another reason to stay conscious while you eat! Stay present to feel how much you have been programmed to eat certain foods, maybe even while you're eating those foods.

After a little detox, you'll begin to see that all kinds of food you previously thought were bland now taste good. Cucumbers can be sweet! Even lettuce is a bit sweet. Compared to 96 ounces of soda, though, they taste bland. So you will need to detox your taste buds as well as detoxing your habits.

This might take a little while, but after you've detoxed your habits and taste buds, you'll be able to choose what you eat way more often than you do now. Right now you are a bit like a lab rat being led around to eat what benefits the people selling you food. You're not quite eating for your own health, vitality, self-esteem, and longevity. You're not even eating for your wallet: junk food gets expensive after a while.

Whenever possible, the NLM is put together in ways that make it work through means other than willpower, to give you the best chance at long-term success. But on some aspects—and junk food is definitely one—you just have to put your foot down. Say to yourself, "I might lose a few battles over the next few months but I will win the war for my health, vitality, family, and future." You don't need to be perfect, and you don't need to kick your own ass about this. As far as I can tell, both of those will put you back into a position where you want to eat junk food and eat to give yourself a little chemical high to stop the self-inflicted pain of the "failure." No one can be perfect once and for all. You simply need to do better than you did yesterday, more often than not.

There will almost certainly be days where everything will fall apart. Cool, no big problem. That is part of the rule, not the exception. Don't beat yourself into giving up on yourself! You just have to get there. You don't have to get there on anyone else's schedule. Don't compare your worst days to someone else's best five minutes, digitally enhanced on social media. Just do enough to reach your targets, your goals, and your aim. You are worth it; don't give up.

Don't ever give up on yourself.

Sleep

People seem to think sleep is a waste of time. This is a very dangerous idea. Over time insufficient sleep will damage your health and vitality and will impair your ability to reach your long-term goals. There are reasons to sleep fewer hours to accomplish a specific short-term goal but consider the long-term effects on your health if you make it a lifestyle.

Mostly, I want you to consider this: What happens to your diet when you aren't sleeping well? Do you automatically reach for bone broth (that you've taken the time to make for yourself), kale, and broccoli, or do you eat junk food, sugar, and caffeine to help stimulate you through the day? Sleep and diet are deeply connected.

We worship the concepts of willpower and force, but we also tend to diminish the usefulness of sleep, as if a really great human being needs no sleep at all. I'd like to shift that perception for you. Going without sleep long term is not a recipe for success, health, strength, or even an indicator of grit or toughness. People need different amounts of sleep. It is possible to change that on some level but ultimately the bill will come due. If you do not get sufficient sleep, you're paying the cost by not getting what you need in terms of your long-term health.

If you want to be healthy, vital, and energetic and maintain the weight you desire, you will need to address your sleep. How much you sleep is important, but how well you sleep is equally if not more important. Start by keeping a little, no-pressure journal.

Ask yourself these questions each day and track your answers:

- How long did you sleep last night?

- How well did you sleep?

- How do you feel today?

- How did you function today?

- Is there anything obvious you can do to make your sleep better?

In popular media, we see these amazing fitness models and well-developed actors and actresses who are totally ripped. But we don't see that, for many of them, a huge chunk of their work is done by sleeping 10 to 12 hours a day.

This whole game is about making the most out of all of your resources in order to accomplish what is most important to you in this short life that we have. Sleep is one of those resources.

Objections to being healthy and vital

This might seem counterintuitive. Why would anyone object to being vital and healthy?

Human nature can indeed be baffling and seemingly illogical. Let's start with the obvious answer to this question: They don't want to have to do something. For example, a person who was constantly belittled as a child by their parents may generally think they cannot function well enough to lead reasonable lives so they self-sabotage. They believe they can't keep a job because they were told that. It's not too far of a stretch to consider that they may reach for food that may make them sick and incapable. They don't do this consciously; it's a consequence of their early learning and the ways they took those terrible lessons into their identities. It's easier to be sick and tired than admit to themselves they feel inferior, so they act in ways to protect them from seeing their true selves.

Other people want to get attention. They learned as children that being ill was a way to get what they needed from their caregivers and over time it became their way of living. They learned that the path to love and affection was by being broken, sick, and in pain so this programming increased those behaviors. They need to learn that getting love and affection for doing things well is far more life-affirming, healthy, and sustainable. Plus, and most importantly, you can never truly get to know yourself if you try to meet your needs this way. Take the chance, be you!

This third group thinks a healthy lifestyle can't be done by them. Sure, it works for other people but it's never worked for them. "What is this crap you're selling?" they may say, every time a possibility for change presents itself. They've tried "everything," they tell themselves and it's all failed to work. Trust me, I know the feeling! But please hear this: you haven't tried everything.

This is all about realizing that on some level you are getting a benefit out of eating poorly, and not doing what you know will lead to greater health and vitality. What is your payoff? Almost no one wants to answer this question, not even privately to themselves because it can be painful to uncover your own unconscious motivations.

Whether this is your specific issue or not, there are treasures unknown to you on the other side of being honest with yourself. Health and vitality are the kind of wealth people don't really understand until it's threatened and they're fighting for it. Be honest with yourself in a kind but decisive way. What negative behaviors give you a payoff that is detrimental to your health, vitality, and diet? Look at them closely, see them for what they are, and decide for yourself a life-building way to get those same needs met. Make a plan—any plan for now—and then execute step one. After step one, reinforce it with thoughts, emotions, and your use of your body to lead you where you want to go.

Create the best you that you can be. Start here and start now; you as you are right now can do this. This is another area that might be quite useful to work on with a professional. They can help you see what you are missing.

Hopefully, application of some of these ideas will help you get over the hump or help you find the missing piece of the equation. Get help if you need it, and don't give up until you have found the answer that works for you.